ANAESTHESIA AND RESUSCITATION:

A manual for medical students

T0334892

Anaesthesia and Resuscitation: a manual for medical students

EDITED BY R. A. GORDON

SECOND EDITION

UNIVERSITY OF TORONTO PRESS

First edition
© University of Toronto Press 1967

Second edition
© University of Toronto Press 1973
Toronto and Buffalo
Reprinted 2017
ISBN 978-0-8020-2097-0 (paper)
LC 67-94389

Preface

The development of modern surgical treatment dates from the introduction of surgical anaesthesia in 1846. Before that time it was seldom that a surgeon had the temerity to invade the cavities of the body, and rarely did patients survive such assaults. For the most part surgery consisted of the amputation of extremities, the drainage of abscesses, and the dressing of wounds. The relief of pain and the production of muscular relaxation provided by the early anaesthetists made possible more precise and leisurely surgery, and at a very early stage enabled the surgeon to explore and operate upon the viscera of the abdomen. Operations within the thorax, the cranial vault, and the airway eventually became possible as knowledge accumulated concerning the physiological disturbances produced by disease of the organs in these regions, and as anaesthetists developed the knowledge and techniques to control these disturbances and the effects of surgical intervention in these areas.

The modern anaesthetist must be a competent physician, equipped by training and experience to recognize and to correct or control the deviations from normal metabolic and homeostatic function which result from pathological processes and surgical intervention. He must be a competent clinical pharmacologist with a nice appreciation of the effects of the potentially lethal drugs which are his armamentarium, and of the variations in these effects produced by abnormal body function. He must stand prepared on the instant to deal with the unusual or the unexpected effects of drugs or surgery. Because of his experience with similar situations in the operating room and because of his command of special techniques, he has become a recognized consultant in problems of ventilation, obstruction of the airway, overdosage of hypnotic and narcotic drugs, resuscitation, and the control of pain.

As in most fields of medical practice many things in anaesthesia are done on an empirical basis and the unanswered questions are legion. The specialty is dynamic and moving, and today's dogma may become tomorrow's error. It is our hope that this volume will provide the student with a firm foundation on which he may build in the future, if he will, a wider knowledge of the boundless realm of anaesthesiology.

PREFACE TO SECOND EDITION

The continuing demand for this manual suggests to the editor and to the authors that it is fulfilling a useful purpose, and hopefully that purpose for which it was designed. Reference is made in the Preface to the First Edition to the rate of change associated with medical knowledge and dogma. Such change accumulated during the six years since the publication of the first edition has dictated a moderate revision of the text. The new edition is published in the hope that it will continue to provide for the medical student a concise discussion of basic information in the field of Anaesthesia and Resuscitation.

R.A. GORDON

Contents

Contributors

R.A. GORDON, C.D., B.SC., M.D., F.R.C.P.(C), F.F.A.R.C.S., Hon.
F.F.A.R.C.S. (Editor)
Professor and Chairman, Department of Anaesthesia, University of
of Toronto
Anaesthetist-in-Chief, Toronto General Hospital

J.M.R. CAMPBELL, M.B., CH.B., F.R.C.P.(C)
Associate Professor, Department of Anaesthesia, University of
Toronto
Anaesthetist-in-Chief, Toronto Western Hospital

JONE CHANG, M.D., F.R.C.P.(C)
Clinical Associate Professor, Department of Anaesthesiology,
University of British Columbia

H.B.F. FAIRLEY, M.B., CH.B., F.R.C.P.(C), F.F.A.R.C.S.
Professor and Vice Chairman, Department of Anaesthesiology,
University of California, San Francisco
Chief of Anaesthesia, San Francisco General Hospital

E.A. GAIN, M.D., F.R.C.P.(C)
Professor and Head, Department of Anaesthesia, University of
Alberta

R.G.B. GILBERT, M.B., CH.B., F.R.C.P.(C), F.F.A.R.C.S.
Anaesthetist, Montreal Neurological Hospital
Anaesthetist, Montreal Chest Hospital Centre

H.B. GRAVES, B.A., M.D., C.M., F.R.C.P.(C)
Clinical Associate Professor of Anaesthesiology, Faculty of
Medicine, University of British Columbia
Associate Director, Department of Anaesthesiology, Vancouver
General Hospital

ANDRÉ JACQUES, C.D., M.D., F.R.C.P.(C), F.F.A.R.C.S.
Anaesthetist-in-Chief, Hôtel Dieu de Québec, Québec

T.J. MCCAUGHEY, M.B., B.CH., F.R.C.P.(C)
Professor, Department of Anaesthesia, McGill University
Director, Department of Anaesthesia, Montreal General Hospital

PAUL E. OTTON, M.D., F.R.C.P.(C)
Associate Professor, Department of Anaesthesia, McGill University
Anaesthetist Royal Victoria Hospital, Montreal

GORDON R. SELLERY, M.D., DIP.ANAES.(Tor.), F.R.C.P.(C)
Clinical Assistant Professor, Department of Anaesthesia, University
of Western Ontario
Anaesthetist-in-Chief, Victoria General Hospital, London, Ontario

W.E. SPOEREL, M.D., F.R.C.P.(C)
Professor and Chairman, Department of Anaesthesia, University of
Western Ontario
Anaesthetist-in-Chief, University Hospital, London, Ontario

CARL C. STODDARD, M.D.
Professor, Department of Anaesthesia, Dalhousie University
Medical School

S.L. VANDEWATER, M.D., F.R.C.P.(C)
Professor, Department of Anaesthesiology, Queen's University.

G.M. WYANT, F.R.C.P.(C), F.F.A.R.C.S.
Professor and Head, Department of Anaesthesia, University of Saskatchewan

ANAESTHESIA AND RESUSCITATION:

A manual for medical students

R.G.B. GILBERT

1
Anaesthesia in relation to surgery

A surgical operation should be an example of teamwork in which the surgeon, anaesthetist, assistant, and nurses all work together, each appreciative of the others' problems. The anaesthetic, of whatever type, should be a not too unpleasant interlude in the hospital experience.

SURGICAL REQUIREMENTS

The anaesthetic selected should be that which will best permit the surgeon to perform the task before him, subject to its suitability to the condition of the patient. The agent and techniques used should be those least likely to produce complications or to interfere with the physiological equilibrium.

Surgical anaesthesia may be considered to have three components. These are hypnosis, analgesia, and muscle relaxation. The anaesthetist should be able to develop each separately, according to the surgical requirements. Neglect of these considerations may result in technical difficulties for the surgeon, possibly in the initiation of reflex disturbances of the homeostatic mechanisms, or even in operative shock. The following are *examples* of special considerations related to the type and site of the surgical operation.

1 *Abdominal surgery* To facilitate surgery and to avoid traction reflexes, there must be not only good analgesia but also adequate

relaxation. Both can be obtained by light general anaesthesia coupled with the use of relaxant drugs or by some form of regional anaesthesia. The older practice of obtaining such relaxation by deep general anaesthesia is associated with disturbances of ventilation and cardiovascular function, which are no longer acceptable. The prior placement of a gastric suction tube is mandatory in most abdominal surgery, but is *not* complete insurance against the aspiration of stomach contents, especially in cases of intestinal obstruction.

2 *Thoracic surgery* To ensure perfect ventilation in the face of a surgical pneumothorax, controlled respiration is necessary. This is achieved by using endotracheal anaesthesia, relaxant drugs and, frequently, an automatic ventilator.

3 *Surgery of the extremities* usually does not demand marked muscle relaxation. Adequate analgesia can be obtained by either light general anaesthesia or a regional technique. The light general anaesthesia will, in addition, produce a hypnotic element.

4 *Paediatric surgery* The surgical requirements are similar to those in the adult, but to obtain them the use of scaled-down equipment is necessary and special attention must be given to infant physiology and anatomy.

5 *Special types of surgery* such as neurosurgery, cardiac surgery, ophthalmic surgery, and obstetrics demand special consideration for their own specific requirements.

Endotracheal Anaesthesia
With some types of surgery, endotracheal anaesthesia may be required or may have certain advantages.
1 General anaesthesia maintained through a tracheal tube, with the cuff inflated or suitably packed off, prevents aspiration of foreign material during ear, nose, and throat surgery.
2 Endotracheal anaesthesia is obligatory for efficient 'controlled ventilation.'
3 The technique forms an additional precautionary measure during abdominal surgery under general anaesthesia, when there is always a possibility of aspiration. When respiration has to be assisted under

this and similar circumstances, the method removes the danger of inflating the stomach.

4 The use of endotracheal anaesthesia permits the anaesthetist to be remote from the operative site when he would otherwise obstruct the field.

5 Endotracheal anaesthesia permits a light plane of anaesthesia to be maintained for long periods without laryngeal spasm which might otherwise occur.

Intravenous Therapy
In all but minor cases an intravenous infusion must be started prior to operation, so that necessary fluids, blood, or drugs may be given.

Suction
Suction should always be available, but it will be needed especially following operations within the oropharynx and nasopharynx.

Regional Anaesthesia
Regional anaesthesia may be selected as the most appropriate method for the patient. A discussion of regional methods of anaesthesia will be found in chapter 6.

THE INFLUENCE OF OPERATIVE POSITION

The operative position of the patient requires special attention by the anaesthetist. In some operative positions the use of a tracheal tube provides the best method of assisting the patient's respiration, besides allowing the anaesthetist to be at a distance from the operative field, as mentioned before.

In certain operative postures such as the Trendelenburg, lateral, prone and lithotomy positions, respiration is likely to be embarrassed. Ventilation must be assisted to prevent respiratory acidosis. The depression of respiration is increased by deepening the plane of anaesthesia or increasing the relaxation produced by relaxant drugs. Patients under regional anaesthesia who are sedated or whose intercostal and abdominal muscles are paralysed by the regional block may present a similar problem.

The prone position requires even more consideration, as some form of support must be devised to leave the abdomen and lower thorax free for respiratory excursions. At the same time, in this position, the inferior vena cava may be compressed, leading to diminished diastolic filling of the heart and an increase in venous pressure below the compression.

In general, anaesthetic drugs cause vasodilatation and depress the circulation. Under this circumstance, rough handling of the patient, postural changes, a foot-down tilt, or the sitting position may result in a fall in blood pressure. Careful observation of the vital signs is imperative during anaesthesia, and particular attention must be paid to them following changes in posture. Any changes must be noted in the early stages before they assume grave proportions. Means should be available to assist the ventilation and to support the circulation.

The operative position of the patient presents other important features. An anaesthetized subject who is probably unconscious and relaxed cannot respond to traction on nerve roots or pressure over superficial nerves. It is therefore essential that he be protected. Special care must be taken to avoid any injuries – for example, to the brachial plexus and the ulnar, radial, and external popliteal nerves. During lengthy operations, pressure sores may develop. The possible areas where they might occur should be borne in mind and steps taken to prevent them.

As a general rule, the operative position of the patient should be that in which the surgeon can best perform his work. It should be possible for the anaesthetist to compensate for the adverse effects of deviation from the more physiological postures.

ANDRÉ JACQUES

2
Evaluation of the patient
before anaesthesia

The anaesthetist's care of the patient will be based on an assessment of physical and emotional status and on the pharmacological and therapeutic history. It is therefore important to obtain a concise but precise history in order to learn pertinent facts about the patient that will make possible the evaluation of his general state and his susceptibilities. These facts should include (*a*) history of constitutional diseases, (*b*) previous surgical and anaesthetic experience, (*c*) previous use of drugs, and (*d*) the specific reasons for surgery and problems related to these.

CONSTITUTIONAL DISEASES

An appropriate history complemented by physical examination will provide information to permit the anaesthetist to take positive action to correct or control concomitant abnormalities detected in heart, lung, kidney, and other systems. The management of the patient during anaesthesia will be modified by these factors.

Cardiac Problems
Pre-existing heart disease predisposes to arrhythmia, congestive failure and cardiac arrest, during and after anaesthesia. Many of the stress situations known to be associated with cardiac standstill may be well tolerated by the normal heart. It is different in the diseased

heart, however. Cardiac reserve is decreased in the presence of myocardial damage, chronic hypoxia, valvular disease and prolonged heart strain. Sudden appearance of hypotension renders the patient vulnerable to cardiac arrest. Four commonly encountered problems serve as examples of the importance of cardiac status.

Mitral stenosis Patients with mitral stenosis can tolerate only minimal amounts of anaesthetic agents.

Myocardial infarction can be ancient, recent, or repeating. The risk of an operation performed after a recent myocardial infarction is greatly increased. Myocardial infarction is often misdiagnosed as perforation of a peptic ulcer or as cholecystitis.

Auricular flutter and fibrillation These pathological conditions are accompanied by sudden changes in pulse rate and by postoperative hypotension.

Stokes-Adams syndrome Atropine suphate is often effective in increasing pulse rate. The use of a pacemaker must be considered.

Cardiac problems should not deny a patient imperative life-saving surgery as dictated by such things as acute massive haemorrhage, acute cardiac tamponade, strangulated hernia, perforation of a viscus, acute appendicitis, torsion of an ovarian cyst, mechanical obstruction of the intestine, acute gangrenous or suppurative cholecystitis, or peripheral embolism, for example. Cardiac patients, in fact, are given a more secure environment than in their ordinary lives when all means of preventing and overcoming apprehension, hypoxia, hypotension, and circulatory overload are made available to them; but it is important that the anaesthetist should recognize the problem.

Respiratory Problems
Pulmonary emphysema and pulmonary sclerosis call for adequate ventilation to overcome poor alveolar exchange and for repeated bronchial aspiration to evacuate secretions. Mechanical ventilators may be life-saving in the postoperative period. Pulmonary emphysema contraindicates the use of mechanical ventilation with negative pressure.

Bronchial asthma precludes the use of drugs such as morphine, thiobarbiturates, and cyclopropane. These drugs have a cholinergic effect and can increase the existing bronchospasm to a degree which may prove fatal.

Patients with indications of respiratory failure from any cause require special attention to their ventilation (Chapter 8).

Renal Problems

There is close association of renal problems with hypotension, cardiac lesions, diabetes, and electrolyte imbalance.

Other Systemic Problems

Diabetes Diabetics are sensitive to ganglionic blocking agents and to tranquillizers. For emergency operation, when the patient's diabetes is not controlled but when there is no ketonuria, 50 to 100 gm of glucose with 25 units of insulin should be given before operation. For emergency operation when ketonuria is present, 100 gm of glucose in 10 per cent solution with 100 units of insulin should be run into a vein until the urine becomes free from diacetic acid. There is real danger of vomiting during induction of anaesthesia in the diabetic with ketosis. Diabetic patients sometimes develop a syndrome simulating an acute abdomen. Hexamethonium and tranquillizers may enhance the action of insulin and cause severe hypoglycaemia. Hypoglycaemia can develop during an operation and is characterized by sweating, pallor, tachycardia, and dilated pupils; it should be treated by intravenous glucose 25 per cent followed by a 5 per cent solution and 25 to 50 units of insulin. Hypoglycaemic coma may be the cause of delayed return of consciousness.

Myasthenia Gravis Mild cases of myasthenia gravis which might be overlooked can cause anaesthetic difficulties. The serum potassium should be estimated, as hypokalaemia aggravates myasthenia. For premedication, preference should be given to meperidine (Demerol) and atropine; opiates and barbiturates should be avoided. The non-depolarizing relaxants are contraindicated, and it must be remembered that decamethonium may act as a non-depolarizer in this disease. Succinylcholine is the preferred relaxant, but this too must be given as sparingly as possible. In carcinomatous neuropathy, especially in carcinoma of the bronchus, there may be a myasthenic response of the motor end-plates and a consequent abnormal behaviour towards relaxants. Neostigmine or edrophonium may be given intravenously with care either during or after operation if respiration is peripherally depressed. Tracheobronchial aspiration must be performed frequently and efficiently.

Hyperthyroidism There can be exacerbation of thyrotoxicosis before or during surgery (hypertension, high systolic pressure, low diastolic pressure, tachycardia, flushing of the skin, fast capillary pulse, 'water hammer' pulse). The crisis can be overcome with an appropriate dose of morphine or a therapeutic spinal or peridural analgesia or by a dose of trimethaphan camphor-sulfonate (Arfonad).

Hypothyroidism Dosage of depressant drugs should be decreased. There is sensitivity to narcotics and hypnotics. The cough reflex is obtunded. Tracheobronchial hypersecretions are possibly present in most cases.

Phaeochromocytoma Sudden changes in blood pressure level can be treated either by phentolamine (Rogitine) against hypertension or by metaraminol (Aramine) against hypotension. Cyclopropane anaesthesia is not advisable.

Haemophilia The patient should be asked about his propensity to bleed after minor injuries.

Porphyria contraindicates the use of barbiturates.

Paraplegia contraindicates cyclopropane and ether. Preference should be given to halothane and spinal analgesia.

Glaucoma contraindicates the use of atropine.

It also goes without saying that the anaesthetist must take note of any abnormality of size, weight, colour, degree of nutrition and hydration, all of which may indicate problems requiring special consideration in management of anaesthesia.

PREVIOUS ANAESTHETIC AND SURGICAL EXPERIENCES

What type of anaesthesia and surgery has the patient previously been subjected to? Was the procedure uneventful or was it stormy with atelectasis, phlebothrombosis, or pulmonary embolism? Is the patient allergic to certain anaesthetics? Has he any history of jaundice?

Previous Use of Drugs

It is necessary to inquire about the drug habits and the possible allergic reactions of a patient who is to undergo an operation, because the use of certain drugs introduces a relatively unfamiliar hazard.

Tranquillizers Used at random by many people who strive for an unattainable goal called serenity, the tranquillizers are not devoid of side-effects which may become manifest at the time of surgery and anaesthesia and add a further burden. Rauwolfia and its alkaloids and phenothiazine derivatives may cause severe hypotension at the time of anaesthesia and operation. The hypotension may occur at any time after induction of anaesthesia is started and can persist for several days after operation. The effect of the rauwolfia derivatives persists for about ten days after the administration of these drugs is discontinued. Atropine sulphate has proved to be a clinically effective antagonist.

Furthermore, tranquillizers, and especially phenothiazine derivatives, can initiate an extrapyramidal syndrome, may cause jaundice, or produce leucopenia and agranulocytosis, reducing resistance to disease so much that the pneumonia patient, for example, will need larger doses of antibiotics and the chronic cardiac patient more frequently develops decompensation. In tranquillized diabetics, coma is more precipitous and more profound. Patients who are bedfast and who receive tranquillizing drugs frequently develop marked trophic ulcers of the heels which in turn are recalcitrant to therapy. Thus it appears that tranquillizers, to some extent at least, reduce the ability to cope with stressful physiological situations.

Tranquillizers potentiate the action of thiobarbiturates and opiates. Rauwolfia lowers the serotonin content of platelets. Patients with phaeochromocytoma may be unusually susceptible to the hypotensive effects of phenothiazine derivatives.

Adrenocortical hormones The administration of adrenocortical hormones should be continued carefully or larger doses should be administered during the period of surgical treatment when a patient has been receiving such hormones up to the time of the operation, or at any time in the last five years. To deprive a patient of this drug, even unwittingly, may leave him with unreactive or exhausted adrenal glands and inability to respond well to surgical stress. Such patients may suffer potassium imbalance.

Anticoagulants More and more patients are receiving anticoagulants; heparin is antagonized by protamine sulphate and blood transfusions. Dicoumarin and coumarin derivatives and indandione compounds are antagonized by vitamin K_1. A stubborn prothrombin deficiency that cannot be corrected by the slow administration of vitamin K_1 further increases the surgical risk.

Quinidine The use of quinidine implies the presence of cardiovascular disease. Quinidine is a depressant to skeletal muscle and antagonizes the muscle contraction produced by acetylcholine or neostigmine. It may initiate complications if a muscular relaxant is administered at the time of operation.

Digitalis also implies the presence of cardiovascular disease. Digitalis antagonizes heparin pharmacologically. Digitalis toxicity may become a clinical problem if hypokalaemia develops during the postoperative period.

Mercurial diuretics and chlorothiazide The urinary electrolyte pattern is similar with both these diuretics. Changes in potassium balance are important, and with diuretic doses of chlorothiazide, potassium excretion is increased and hypokalaemia frequently occurs. Chlorothiazide has been reported to enhance the hypotensive effects of various agents used in the treatment of hypertension. Hypokalaemia may precipitate digitalis intoxication.

Antibiotics It should be known if the patient has suffered untoward side-effects after the administration of antibiotics. The widespread use of these drugs has caused allergic reactions in some cases. The intestinal flora can be disturbed. Streptomycin, neomycin, and kanamycin potentiate myoneural block, when used intraperitoneally.

Alcohol Chronic alcoholics are prone to fatty embolism, to a low level of serum magnesium, and to a fall of eosinophil count. Shock and aldosterone also produce hypomagnesaemia. Alcoholism can be a factor in precipitating hepatic coma. Alcohol addicts may require large doses of barbiturates and volatile anaesthetics, in comparison to normal individuals.

Ganglionic blocking agents It is worth remembering the undesirable side-effects of these agents. These are dry mouth, paralysis of the iris and ciliary muscles, paralytic ileus, and retention of urine.

Narcotics and hypnotics Use of these drugs suggests the possible presence of allergy. Habituation and addiction presuppose increase of dosage in the postoperative period.

Radiation therapy can be a cause of anaemia, leucopenia, lowered antibodies, and lowered plasma cholinesterase.

Cancer chemotherapy Whether cancer therapy consists of general cell poisons, antimetabolites, alternation of hormonal balance, or specific cell poisons, their administration will affect the patient's physiological status, lower resistance to stress and cause changes in red and white blood cells and platelets.

REFERENCES

DOBKIN, A.B.; HARLAND, J.H.; & FEDORUK, S. Comparison of the Cardiovascular Effects of Halothane and Halothane-Diethyl-Ether Azeotrope in Dogs. Anesthesiology. *21*: 13 (1960)

RALSTON, L.S. Medical Evaluation of the Patient before Operation. Post-Graduate Medicine. *26*: 484 (1959)

RAPHAEL, S.S., LYNCH, M.J.; SPARE, P.D.; & MELLOR, L.D. Further Studies in Chronic Alcoholism. Canadian Medical Association Journal. *82*: 16 (1960)

SHAW, C.C. & FELTS, P.W. Treacherous Tranquilizers. Anesthesia and Analgesia. *38*: 319 (1959)

ANDRÉ JACQUES

3
Preanaesthetic medication

Along with the preanaesthetic visit and evaluation of the patient's problems, preanaesthetic medication is another step towards uneventful anaesthetic management. Essentially, premedication is the use of drugs to prepare the patient for the administration of anaesthetics.

OBJECTIVES

Premedication is determined in relation to the surgical operation (magnitude, duration, site), and its objectives are slightly different if it is used before general anaesthesia or before local, regional, or spinal analgesia. It is administered for the following reasons:

1 *Before general anaesthesia* for its action on psychic activity. (*a*) *Action on psychic activity*; (i) to allay fear, anxiety, and apprehension, whether manifested by mere dread, or by panic (not forgetting feigned swagger); (ii) to induce a state of calm, euphoria, mental relaxation, or semi-somnolence by reducing consciousness and cortical activity, to allow the patient happily to face the weird spectacle of the operating room; (iii) to maintain the patient (ideally) in an obtunded state of consciousness and alertness: a complete preanaesthetic loss of consciousness carries the menace of respiratory obstruction and hypoxia. (*b*) *Action on reflex activity*: to promote induction of anaesthesia devoid of incidents and acci-

dents caused by neurovegetative reflexes such as nausea, eructation, vomiting, cardiac arrhythmias, respiratory disturbances, laryngeal and bronchial spasm, salivary and tracheobronchial hypersecretions. (c) *Action on metabolic activity*: to reduce the necessary doses of anaesthetics, to allow a calm awakening, and a quiet postanaesthetic period.

2 *Before local, regional and spinal analgesia* (a) to suppress individual susceptibility and preoperative and postoperative anxiety; to obtund sensibility to touch and pressure; to elevate the threshold of pain; (b) to potentiate the local anaesthetic action; (c) to overcome reactions to toxicity and shock; (d) to allow operations of long duration.

HISTORICAL ASPECTS

In 1861, Pitha of Vienna promoted the use of an enema containing 1 gm of belladonna extract before induction of anaesthesia. Morphia was the first drug to be used for preanaesthetic sedation. In 1869, Claude Bernard (Leçons sur les anaesthésique et l'asphyxie, J.B. Baillière, ed., Paris, 1875) experimented on animals with morphia before the inhalation of chloroform. In 1870, Clover was prescribing a tablespoon of brandy (spiritus vini gallici) before the administration of chloroform. In 1883, Dastre and Morat (Les Anesthésiques, Masson, ed., Paris, 1890) were relying on the combined administration of morphia and atropine. In 1895, Langlois and Maurange (Comptes Rendus de l'Académie des Sciences, 1895, 121, 263) advised on the use of morphia and sparteine. In 1906, Gauss (Medical Klinik, 1906, 2, 136) was using morphia-scopolamine.

DRUGS USED FOR PREANAESTHETIC MEDICATION

1 *Central analgesics* Morphia, its derivatives and substitutes: (a) to establish a preanaesthetic state; (b) to allay agitation during induction of anaesthesia; (c) to diminish the total dose of anaesthetics required; (d) to obtain calm recovery.

In emergency surgery, opiates and narcotic substitutes should be administered in minimum doses or not at all. Some patients will already have received narcotics by the subcutaneous or intramuscular route on their way to hospital. Hypotension will probably have prevented the drug from taking full effect. Once normal circulation is re-established, the patient may fall into coma and present a diagnostic dilemma, if he happens to have suffered a head injury or is a diabetic or an alcoholic. Narcotics should not be administered to ambulatory patients, nor should they be injected into patients who demonstrate hypoventilation from any cause or who are unconscious. Narcotics can be given slowly by the intravenous route. Reaction to pain must not be confused with excitement and agitation associated with hypoxia. As a general rule, narcotics should not be administered to infants and children; if they are, it must be with great caution and care in dosage and with immediate cardiorespiratory supervision.

2 *Anticholinergics* atropine, scopolamine, and their derivatives: (*a*) to obviate cardiac arrhythmias; (*b*) to abolish salivary and tracheobronchial hypersecretions.

3 *Hypnotics* Barbiturates, non-barbiturates. Hypnotics will induce sleep. They may cause agitation in a patient who has pain.

4 *Antihistamines* (*a*) to promote somnolence; (*b*) to overcome allergic reaction to drugs.

5 *Neuroplegics*

6 *Tranquillizers*

7 *Neuroleptataralgesics.*

Dosage of preanaesthetic medication will vary according to: (*a*) the type of anaesthesia – general, local, regional, or spinal; (*b*) the type of anaesthetic agent; (*c*) the type and location of surgical operation, keeping in mind the reflexogenic zones (thoracic, upper abdominal, cervical, and perineal); (*d*) the patient, his age, and his physical status: in children, scopolamine should be preferred to atropine (minimal tachycardia); in geriatrics, scopolamine may cause agitation and hallucination. In considering the patient's physical status one takes note of cardiac disease, pulmonary disease, ethylism, toxicomania, epilepsy, anaemia, shock, hepatic and renal diseases, infection, hyperthyroidism, hypothyroidism, collagen diseases, porphyria, phaechromocytoma, paraplegia.

Tabulations Every anaesthetist seems to have a preference and a motive for a drug or a combination of drugs to be used as preanaesthetic medication. Pertinent tabulations can be found in every manual and textbook on anaesthesia. However, this variety of preferences and tastes must always respect the fundamental principles of human physiology and pharmacology. The following references illustrate some of these tabulations.

REFERENCES

ALLUAUME, R. La Prémédication. Cours pour la préparation au certificat d'études spéciales d'anesthésiologie. 957, tome 2 (1958). Paris: Librairie Arnette

CULLEN, S.C. Anesthesia in General Practice, 4th edition. Preanesthetic Medication. 44 (1954). Chicago: Year Book Publishers

DELAHAYE, G. Prémédications. Cours pour la préparation au certificat d'études spéciales d'anesthésiologie. 157, fascicule 1 (1954). Paris: Librairie Arnette

DRIPPS, ROBERT D.; ECKENHOFF, JAMES E.; & VANDAM, LEROY D. Introduction to Anesthesia. Guides to Preanesthetic Medication. 9 (1957). Philadelphia: W.B. Saunders

KEOWN, KENNETH K. Anesthesia for Surgery of the Heart. Preliminary Medication. 15 (1956). Springfield, Ill.: Charles C. Thomas

KIESEWETTER, WILLIAM B. Pre- and Post-operative Care in Pediatric Surgical Patient. Preanesthetic Medication. 33 (1956). Chicago: Year Book Publishers

LEIGH, M. DIGBY & BELTON, KATHLEEN M.M. Pediatric Anesthesia. 4 (1948). New York: Macmillan

MERCIER, FERNAND. Les bases pharmacodynamiques de la médication préanesthésique. Actualités pharmacologiques. Troisième série: 49 (1951). Paris: Masson

SCHWARTZ, HERMAN; NGAI, S.H.; & PAPPER, E.M. Manual of Anesthesiology. Premedication. 16 (1957). Springfield, Ill.: Charles C. Thomas

W.E. SPOEREL AND G.R. SELLERY

4
General anaesthesia

General anaesthesia involves three basic components; these are hypnosis or loss of consciousness, analgesia or loss of responsiveness to afferent stimuli, and muscle relaxation. Agents used to produce general anaesthesia vary in their capabilities in this regard. The precise mode of action of anaesthetic agents is not known, although a number of theories have been proposed.

All general anaesthetic agents exert their influence on the central nervous system without a change in the chemical structure. Gases and vapours used for inhalation anaesthesia are for the most part eliminated unchanged through the lungs except for small amounts which are metabolized and so release degradation products. Injectable agents are detoxified or rendered inactive by the liver and are excreted unchanged or as metabolic products by the kidneys.

Depression of function of the central nervous system depends on the potency of the particular anaesthetic agent and the concentration of that agent at the site of action. For each inhalational agent there is a minimal alveolar concentration which is just sufficient to obtund a specific stimulus. Therefore, for a specific depth of anaesthesia a known concentration of an agent will have to be administered. Response to anaesthetic drugs varies from patient to patient. Older patients and those in shock due to cardiac insufficiency or hypovolaemia are very sensitive and require relatively small doses while muscular patients may recover quickly after large doses. Tolerance is increased in alcoholic patients and those addicted to opiates and barbiturates.

To understand the means by which the anaesthetist can induce a state of anaesthesia, control the depth of anaesthesia, and effect the recovery of the patient, it is essential to understand the mechanisms involved in the uptake of gases and vapours into the bloodstream, their transport to the central nervous system, and their removal by redistribution within the body and eventual excretion, either by the lungs or kidneys, which will affect the duration of the recovery period.

UPTAKE OF ANAESTHETIC GASES AND VAPOURS

Agents commonly used for inhalation anaesthesia at the present time are listed in Table I and are discussed in detail in a later section of this chapter. Depending on their physical characteristics they are in a gaseous or liquid phase at room temperature and are classified as anaesthetic gases or volatile anaesthetic liquids. The latter must be converted into vapours before they are administered. Anaesthetic gases and vapours behave for practical purposes as inert gases and in the following discussion they will be referred to as gases only.

The anaesthetic breathing apparatus delivers a concentration of an inhalation agent which is selected by the anaesthetist. In the case of volatile agents such as ether, halothane, or methoxyflurane, factors affecting vaporization are important. Thus the temperature of the liquid, vapour pressure, and the surface area exposed will determine the concentration reaching the lungs. Cooling of an agent with a low vapour pressure (e.g. methoxyflurane) due to the loss of heat of vaporization will result in a low inspired concentration in the anaesthetic circuit. Temperature compensated vaporizers (Fluotec®, Pentec®) are valuable to avoid this problem.

The entrance of anaesthetic gases into the lungs, their diffusion into the blood stream and their solubility in blood and tissues are governed by physical laws describing the properties of gases. The application of these laws makes it possible to predict mathematically the effect of inhalation of a known concentration of anaesthetic gas with sufficient accuracy to provide a basis for the conduct of clinical

Table I

Physical and chemical properties of inhalation anaesthetics

Agent	Formula	Boiling point (°C)	Vapour pressure (25 °C)	Blood-gas ratio	Oil/water ratio	Inhaled range	Concentration for anaesthesia maintenance (vol. %)	Flammable
Gases								
Cyclopropane	C_3H_6	−33	90 p.s.i.	0.46	35	5–25	10–15	Yes
Nitrous Oxide	N_2O	−89	800 p.s.i.	0.46	3.1	50–80	50–80 (+ supplement)	No
Volatile liquids								
Ether	$(C_2H_5)_2O$	35	540 mm Hg	15	3.2	3–10	3–5	Yes
Trichlorethylene	$C_2H\,Cl_3$	87	70 mm Hg	8–10	400	0.7–1.3	0.7	No
Halothane	$C_2F_3\,HBr\,Cl$	50	300 mm Hg	3.6	280	0.5–4	0.8–1.2	No
Methoxyflurane	$CH\,Cl_2CF_2O\,CH_3$	104	25 mm Hg	11–13	400	0.5–1.5	0.4–0.8	No

Note: Modified from Dripps *et al*, Introduction to Anesthesia, Philadelphia, Saunders (1961)

anaesthesia. An understanding of the relationship between the inhaled concentration of an anaesthetic gas and the tension in the tissues of the central nervous system requires knowledge of the following basic principles:

1 The addition of an anaesthetic gas to the inhaled atmosphere will change the composition of the alveolar gases. Dalton's law states: *In a mixture of gases each exerts its own pressure independent of other gases; the total pressure is the sum of the partial pressures.* The addition of an anaesthetic gas will cause a corresponding reduction in the tension of oxygen and nitrogen.

2 The rate of diffusion of an anaesthetic gas from the alveoli into the blood is proportional to the gradient of concentration (Fick's Law). With equal concentrations the rate of diffusion is inversely proportional to the square root of the molecular weight (Graham's Law). Most anaesthetic gases will diffuse more slowly than oxygen or carbon dioxide, but the rate of diffusion can be increased by increasing the diffusion gradient, i.e., the inhaled concentration.

3 Each alveolus and its capillary network represents an interphase between air and blood. Gas will dissolve in blood until the tension of the gas is equal in air and blood (Henry's Law). The volume of gas in solution required to equilibrate with the volume of gas in the alveolus at the same tension is expressed as blood-gas ratio, blood-gas solubility coefficient or partition coefficient (Table 1). This coefficient presents a key for the understanding of some important properties of anaesthetic gases.

4 Blood and tissues contain two principal solvents, water and lipoids. Since all anaesthetic gases have a high lipoid solubility (Table 1, oil-water ratio), the lipoid content of blood and tissues will influence the volume of gas dissolved. The tissue-blood ratio will be greater than one for most tissues and this will influence the establishment of an equilibrium of gas tension between blood and tissues. Fat tissue has an immense capacity to absorb anaesthetic gases.

A known concentration of anaesthetic gas is delivered to the lungs by the anaesthetic system. The concentration in the alveoli will now depend on pulmonary ventilation and the rate at which the agent leaves the alveoli to enter the circulation. As ventilation increases, the alveolar concentration will increase to closely approximate the concentration in the anaesthetic circuit. If large amounts of the agent are taken up by the pulmonary circulation due either to a high solubility in blood or to a high blood flow, the alveolar concentration will be low. Thus the alveolar tension will be low. If the alveolar tension is low the brain tension will also be low, even though there may be a large amount of anaesthetic dissolved in the blood and tissues.

Therefore, theoretically one increases the speed of induction of anaesthesia by having a high inspired concentration, increased pulmonary ventilation, a very insoluble agent and a low cardiac output. When all physiological factors in the patient are kept constant, a gas with a low blood-gas coefficient (i.e. very insoluble) such as nitrous oxide or cyclopropane will reach equilibrium rapidly, so that the alveolar and brain tension will reach a high level quickly, thus increasing the speed of induction. Halothane is intermediate in solubility while ether and methoxyflurane are very soluble, thus ensuring a very slow induction of anaesthesia.

If anaesthesia were to be induced by having the patient inhale gas at the tension required for the maintenance of surgical anaesthesia, induction would be very slow and with some agents, never complete (Fig. 1). The anaesthetist will overcome this problem by using tensions considerably higher than those required for maintenance. Often potentially lethal concentrations are administered to induce anaesthesia rapidly. In this way the tension of the anaesthetic gas required for maintenance of anaesthesia is quickly reached in the central nervous system, although the remainder of the organism is not equilibrated to this tension. When the patient has reached a state of clinical anaesthesia, the inspired concentration is reduced to the level required for maintenance. This method affords rapid induction of anaesthesia with cyclopropane and halothane. When ether or methoxyflurane are used a rapid induction is not possible, since high concentrations cannot be used for induction. Ether vapour is irritating to mucous membrane while methoxyflurane, with a boiling point of 104° C, does not produce sufficient vapour tension at room temperature.

The depth of anaesthesia corresponds to the tension of an anaes-

% INSPIRED TENSION

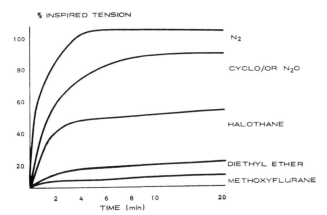

FIGURE 1   Effect of solubility in blood of the inert gas on its alveolar or arterial uptake curve, all physiologic factors remaining constant. Modified from S. Kety, Anesthesiology, 11: 519 (1950)

thetic gas in the brain. The rich blood supply of the brain allows a rapid equilibrium between the arterial and the tissue tension of the anaesthetic; it is, therefore, possible to correlate depth of anaesthesia and arterial tension of an anaesthetic gas.

A rapid equilibration can be expected in all other vital organs (heart, liver, kidneys), which represent 7 to 8 per cent of the body weight and receive 70 per cent of the cardiac output. The mass of the body (92 per cent of body weight) receives only 30 per cent of the total blood flow. With an equal or (in case of fat tissue) much higher capacity to absorb anaesthetic gases, it will take considerably longer to establish an equilibrium between blood and tissue. In fat tissue, with the highest capacity to absorb anaesthetic agents and the lowest blood supply, such equilibrium is probably never obtained.

The figures given in Table II represent the distribution of the cardiac output at rest. If the peripheral blood flow is increased by muscular activity, apprehension or fever, equilibrium is obtained more quickly in parts of the body mass and consequently a larger volume of anaesthetic gas is required to reach the arterial tension

Table II

Blood flow to vital organs and other tissues

	Weight (kg)	Blood flow (ml/100 gm tissue)	Cardiac output (%)
Vital organs			
Brain	1.4	54	13.9
Heart	0.3	85	4.7
Hepatic-portal			
region	2.6	58	27.7
Kidneys	0.3	420	23.3
Other tissues	58.4	3	30.4

Note: Modified from Dripps *et al.*, Introduction to Anesthesia, Philadelphia, Saunders (1961)

necessary to maintain anaesthesia. In conditions of shock and diminished blood volume, the peripheral blood flow is markedly reduced and a much smaller volume of anaesthetic is sufficient to establish an adequate anaesthetic tension.

REDISTRIBUTION OF ANAESTHETICS

If respiration were to be stopped immediately after anaesthesia had been induced or ventilation carried out with a closed breathing system, and if there were no further addition of anaesthetic gas, the arterial tension would fall rapidly and the patient could even regain consciousness, although he had exhaled no anaesthetic agent. This phenomenon is caused by redistribution of the anaesthetic agent from areas where an equilibrium was attained quickly (i.e. the vital organs, notably the brain) to areas with a lower blood flow, where more time is required to establish such equilibrium. The magnitude of the redistribution effect will decrease as anaesthesia is prolonged. There remains, however, a constant loss of anaesthetic gas into fat tissue, which has an almost unlimited capacity for absorption, but receives only 1 to 3 per cent of the cardiac output. Other small losses also occur because of diffusion of the anaesthetic gas into the intestines and through the skin and the tissues exposed to the air by the surgical incision. Hence after the uptake of the large volume of anaesthetic gas required during induction, there will be a gradually decreasing requirement which, after some time, will remain almost constant. A small volume of anaesthetic gas must be supplied continuously throughout the course of anaesthesia to replace this internal loss if an even level of anaesthetic depression is to be maintained.

Clinical application During induction of inhalation anaesthesia, potentially lethal concentrations of anaesthetics are employed. If they are administered too long they will cause respiratory arrest, an event which not only alarms the anaesthetist but also stops the uptake of further anaesthetic. In a healthy patient the redistribution will reduce the arterial tension fast enough to allow the respiratory centre to recover, often without artificial ventilation; respiratory arrest in the course of induction of anaesthesia often has a good outcome if properly managed. But an overdose is much more dangerous in a patient who is very ill or hypovolaemic. Because of the low peripheral blood flow, there is little redistribution, and even with vigorous attempts at resuscitation and elimination of anaesthetic agents through the lungs the arterial tension will be less rapidly reduced.

Elimination of Inhalation Agents
All inhalation anaesthetics exert their effect as inert gases and are eliminated by exhalation. The same physical and physiological factors which determine the uptake also influence the removal from tissues and blood. Gases with a low solubility coefficient will be eliminated more rapidly than those with a high blood-gas ratio. The duration of the anaesthetic will also influence recovery; after a short procedure redistribution and exhalation of the anaesthetic gas will lower the arterial tension quite rapidly, while after a long procedure the large volume of gas stored in the body mass will be released slowly and maintain an arterial tension which may be responsible for prolonged post-anaesthetic depression. Increased alveolar ventilation will hasten recovery. Although the anaesthetic concentration in the blood usually falls to levels allowing the return of consciousness within the first hour after the end of an operation, sub-anaesthetic concentrations are usually present for many hours, and

traces are present for days, presumably because they are released very slowly from fat tissues. These low concentrations may be a factor contributing to the morbidity of the immediate post-anaesthetic period, manifested by drowsiness, nausea, and vomiting, vasomotor instability, and occasional headache. Recent studies with radioactive carbon have shown that agents which were thought to be inert are in part metabolized. Trichlorethylene is metabolized in part to trichloracetic acid, which can be demonstrated in the urine for six to ten days after anaesthesia. Halothane and methoxyflurane form metabolic degradation products which may have an effect on the liver and kidneys respectively.

AGENTS USED FOR INHALATION ANAESTHESIA

The agents listed in Table I are those most commonly used in clinical practice. Many hydrocarbons having anaesthetic properties have been used in the past but have not gained widespread acceptance; others are being investigated (Forane®, Ethrane®). The acceptance of an agent is influenced not only by desirable pharmacological properties but also by surgical requirements which may be unrelated to the patient. The increased use of diathermy and X-ray in the operating room has contributed greatly to a decline in the use of flammable anaesthetic agents.

Agents with a high partition coefficient which cannot be administered in high concentrations (e.g., ether, methoxyflurane), are often described as 'safe.' This only implies that, because of their physical properties, lethal concentrations are more difficult to administer when the patient is breathing spontaneously. Although this minimizes the danger of an overdosage in inexperienced hands, the slow induction and more difficult maintenance introduce other problems which make anaesthesia more unpleasant and perhaps more hazardous for the patient.

Potent agents can be administered safely if accurate flow meters (e.g., cyclopropane) or calibrated vaporizers (e.g., halothane) are used. Nitrous oxide and ethylene are weak anaesthetic agents that can produce only very light surgical anaesthesia in concentrations up to 80 per cent of inspired gas. They must always be used with oxygen and should be supplemented with other anaesthetic agents (see below).

The important physical, chemical and pharmacological properties and some clinical features of agents used for inhalation anaesthesia are listed in Table I. The following short notes outline the history and present usefulness of each agent.

These agents can be divided into two major groups. Those agents which are in the gas phase at room temperature are stored in cylinders and administered as gases. Examples are nitrous oxide, cyclopropane, and ethylene. The latter two agents are used infrequently because they are explosive. The second group consists of substances which are volatile liquids at room temperature and require vaporization for administration to the patient. Over the past ten years there have been many changes in the types of agents used for this purpose. The increased use of diathermy and monitoring equipment in the operating room has meant that explosive agents could not be used. This means that cyclopropane, ethylene, diethyl ether, divinyl ether, and ethyl chloride are no longer being used to any great degree in most Canadian hospitals.

Other agents such as chloroform have toxic side effects which offset their benefits when safer agents are available. At present the commonly used agents with which the student must be familiar are nitrous oxide, halothane, and methoxyflurane. Agents currently under investigation (1973) include Forane and Ethrane. These agents have not yet been released for general clinical use. Ether, cyclopropane, and trichlorethylene may be used in some areas and the student should be aware of these agents.

The Anaesthetic Gases

Nitrous oxide First prepared by Priestley in 1772 and used for anaesthesia by Horace Wells, a dentist who made an unsuccessful attempt in 1844 to introduce its use at the Massachusetts General Hospital in Boston. It is a gas at room temperature, colourless, non-explosive and non-irritating. It is stored as a liquid in cylinders at a pressure of approximately 750 p.s.i. The cylinders are blue in colour and pin-indexed so that a nitrous-oxide cylinder will not fit an oxygen cylinder yoke.

The partial pressure of nitrous oxide in the blood allows it to diffuse into gas containing cavities. This can cause distention of the gastrointestinal tract or cause an enlargement of a lung cyst or other closed air pockets such as a pneumothorax. If a pneumo-encephalogram is done, the inhalation of nitrous oxide can increase intracranial pressure, with serious sequelae. Even when administered with oxygen at a concentration of 75 per cent it will not satisfactorily anaesthetize a healthy patient. Therefore, either intermittent intravenous injections of narcotic or more potent inhalation agents are required to maintain surgical anaesthesia. It has found use, however, in pain relief during labour and delivery, change of burn dressings when mild degrees of analgesia are required without complete anaesthesia. It is universally used as a vehicle in association with oxygen for the vaporization of potent inhalation agents. In many hospitals it is piped in from large tanks to the anaesthetic machine.

Ethylene Has been used in the same manner as nitrous oxide, but it is not used at present because it is highly flammable and creates an explosion hazard.

Cyclopropane Developed initially in 1929 by Lucas and Henderson in Toronto and was popularized by Waters in Madison, Wisconsin. It is a very potent anaesthetic gas allowing rapid induction of anaesthesia but not as potent as the volatile agents, a concentration of 12–15 per cent being required for maintenance. It causes early vasoconstriction resulting in hypertension, a factor that was thought to be useful in the management of the shocked patient. It causes marked respiratory depression so that when deep planes of anaesthesia are achieved without the use of artificial ventilation, marked CO_2 retention occurs.

A closed circuit method is usually used for cyclopropane because it is explosive. This means that cyclopropane is administered at a flow rate of 25 cc to 50 cc per minute along with oxygen at the flow rate required for oxygen consumption. This decreases the chance of explosion because minimal amounts of cyclopropane are exhaled to room air and the expiratory valve is kept closed. However, this still is dangerous as some anaesthetic circuits have small leaks where the gas may escape. Discharges of static electricity produced in the operating room may serve as sources of ignition, and are difficult to control even when the electrical circuits and other electrical features are acceptable.

Volatile Anaesthetic Agents

A liquid anaesthetic agent is transformed into a vapour for inhalation at a speed which depends on its vapour pressure at room temperature. For example, at room temperature the vapour pressure of diethyl ether is 450 mm Hg, that of halothane is 240 mm Hg, and methoxyflurane is 23 mm Hg. It is difficult to vaporize methoxyflurane, so that it depends on its high potency to achieve anaesthesia.

Diethyl ether Usually called 'ether,' was used by W.E. Clark and Crawford Long in 1842. W.T.G. Morton demonstrated its use at the Massachusetts General Hospital in 1846. In the past it was considered to be the safest anaesthetic agent because of its slow action and the stability of the cardiovascular system. At deep levels it provides excellent muscle relaxation. Its disadvantage is that it is explosive. It is also irritating to the respiratory tract during induction. Its use is associated with a high incidence of postoperative nausea and vomiting, and this has also affected its popularity. Ether was the basic anaesthetic agent upon which the classical descriptions of the signs and stages of general anaesthesia were based. These were developed by Snow and by Guedel, who defined and described the signs and stages of anaesthesia in relationship to the character of respiration, eyeball activity, pupillary changes, presence or absence of the eyelid reflexes, swallowing, and vomiting, etc. In the Guedel classification Stage I of anaesthesia lasts from the beginning of anaesthesia to the loss of consciousness, and the patient's reaction to pain is altered so that it is commonly called the stage of analgesia. Stage II is the stage of excitement or delirium and lasts from the loss of consciousness to the onset of a regular pattern of breathing and disappearance of lid reflex. During this stage the patient should not be stimulated. Respiration may be irregular, pupils are often dilated, and the patient may move about and require restraint. It is advisable to pass through this stage quickly by rapidly increasing the inhaled concentration of the anaesthetic. Stage III is the stage of surgical anaesthesia and lasts from the onset of regular breathing to the cessation of respiration. It is divided into four planes, which are usually determined by the amount of intercostal muscle paralysis. In plane I the eyeballs may become eccentrically fixed, whereas in plane II the eyeballs cease to move and become central. Reflex closing of the vocal cords or laryngospasm begins to disappear in plane II and muscular tone lessens. In plane III intercostal activity begins to decrease and the pupils begin to dilate. This is the plane during which most surgical operations are accomplished, as there is moderate muscle relaxation. Plane IV starts with the complete paralysis of intercostal muscles to the cessation of spontaneous respiration. CO_2 accumulation may occur if diaphragmatic activity is not adequate. Stage IV involves complete medullary paralysis and action must be taken to maintain respiratory and circulatory function. This stage should never be entered in a normal safe anaesthetic.

Divinyl ether (Vinethene) was used for short anaesthetics and the induction of anaesthesia followed by ether. The agent is flammable and decomposed by light. It is little used today.

Ethyl chloride Another rapidly acting non-irritating volatile agent used for induction of anaesthesia by the open drop technique. With a boiling point of 12° C., it is a gas at room temperature and must, therefore, be kept in special bottles under a pressure of 40 mm Hg. It has little use for anaesthesia today.

Chloroform was first prepared in 1832 and was first used as an anaesthetic agent by Simpson in 1847. It has toxic effects on the heart and, particularly, on the liver. It is not used at the present time because there are safer agents available.

Trichloroethylene (Trilene) First described by Fisher in 1854 was initially used as a solvent for dry-cleaning. It is a non-explosive anaesthetic that can be used as a supplement to nitrous oxide anaesthesia. It has good analgesic properties but is not a good muscle relaxant. It has a low vapour pressure, so that induction is slow. Owing to stimulation of the pulmonary deflation receptors it produces tachypnoea, which may be managed with narcotics. It cannot be used in the closed or semiclosed circuits as it decomposes in the presence of the soda lime to produce toxic substances (dichloroacetylene) which may damage the central nervous system. In some older anaesthetic machines the circle system could not be used when the trilene vaporizer was in the 'on' position. It is not used much at present, although self-administered trilene analgesia may be helpful in labour.

Halothane (Fluothane) was synthetized by Imperial Chemical Industries in 1951 and introduced clinically by Johnstone in 1956 as a non-flammable, non-irritating, apparently non-toxic, and very potent anaesthetic agent. It has gained widespread popularity and is considered an almost ideal anaesthetic agent by some. Its high potency makes the use of a calibrated vaporizer mandatory. It can be used in the circle system as it does not react with soda lime. The vapour pressure is about 240 mm Hg at room temperature, which is about one half that of ether. Therefore, it can be used by the open drop technique but is very suitable for vaporization in a bubble-through vaporizer (copper kettle) or flow controlled temperature compensated vaporizer (Fluotec).

Halothane is relatively insoluble, so that its alveolar tension can soon approach the inspired halothane tension. Because brain tension is almost the same as alveolar tension, induction of anaesthesia is rapid when compared to more soluble agents such as ether and methoxyflurane.

Respiration is depressed especially with addition of narcotic premedication. It may be necessary to assist ventilation to prevent hypoventilation and CO_2 retention, although hypoventilation is usually a sign of overdosage.

Halothane depresses the myocardium and causes peripheral vasodilatation, which may lead to hypotension. Bradycardia may occur because of a parasympathomimetic action, but this may be reversed with atropine. Halothane also may sensitize the heart to the action of adrenaline, and ventricular extrasystoles may occur when adrenaline is infiltrated to reduce blood loss.

Halothane has no specific action on the kidneys or liver unless as an effect secondary to marked and prolonged hypotension. However, over the past ten years a number of cases of acute hepatic necrosis have occurred following halothane anaesthesia. Even though many factors can lead to postoperative hepatic damage, it is generally conceded that a small number of these cases may be due to specific sensitivity to halothane or to hepatotoxicity of intermediate metabolites of the drug. It is more common after repeated halothane anaesthetics. Therefore, most authorities would agree that halothane should not be used if jaundice, for which no other cause can be found, occurred following a previous anaesthetic. Many anaesthetists do not repeat a halothane anaesthetic within three months of a previous one.

Relaxation of the uterine muscle is another feature, making halothane useful for obstetrical procedures where such relaxation is important. However, this may be harmful because post partum haemorrhage may be more likely to occur. Halothane easily crosses the placental barrier.

The action of the non-depolarizing muscle relaxants is potentiated so that smaller doses are required. Its action on the cerebral blood vessels producing vasodilatation results in an increase in intracranial pressure so that its use in neurosurgical anaesthesia may not be recommended.

Methoxyflurane (Penthrane) An agent recently developed by Abbott Laboratories. Its anaesthetic properties were described by Artusio and Van Poznack in 1960. With a boiling point of 104° C. it has a low vapour pressure of 23 mm Hg. It has a high partition coefficient (very soluble) making induction and recovery slow. It has a peculiar fruity odour and is relatively non-irritating and non-flammable in concentrations used clinically. Next to ether, methoxyflurane provides the greatest degree of muscular relaxation and in contrast to halothane has fairly good analgesic properties.

The effects of methoxyflurane on the body systems are fairly similar to those of halothane in equi-potent doses. However, it has the serious disadvantage that, when administered in rather high concentrations over long periods, some of the drug is metabolized, leaving a fluoride ion residue which is toxic to the kidney. Some patients have developed high output renal failure. This may last for many months or may be fatal. Therefore, it is wise to avoid its use in patients with renal disease and in long operations. It is not very suitable in the very short operations because of its high solubility and, therefore, slow induction (i.e. the operation may be over before the patient is properly asleep!).

INTRAVENOUS ANAESTHETIC AGENTS

Ultra-short-acting barbiturates have gained widespread acceptance for the induction of anaesthesia. Thiopentone, as an example of this group, when injected intravenously is diluted and distributed through the bloodstream. The time required for circulation to the brain determines the speed of onset of anaesthesia since the drug diffuses rapidly into the tissues. Following intravenous injection the blood concentration and tissue concentration rapidly reach a peak. The concentration then falls rapidly and the patient may regain consciousness with a blood level slightly higher than at the onset. The initial reduction in blood concentration is due to redistribution of the drug to the vital areas and to peripheral tissues. Thiopentone has a marked affinity for fat tissue and the blood concentration is slowly reduced by continuous absorption of the drug by fat.

The metabolic destruction of thiopentone occurs mainly in the liver at a rate of about 15 per cent per hour. Less then 1 per cent is excreted unchanged in the urine. The metabolism of the drug can be increased if the patient has been taking barbiturates prior to its use. This increased metabolism is due to enzyme induction, a circumstance in which enzymes are available in the liver to destroy thiopentone because of their initial stimulation by other barbiturates.

The redistribution of the drug represents the predominant means by which quick recovery occurs. With subsequent doses this becomes less efficient and the blood level will remain higher after each injection. Consequently the anaesthetic depression will last longer after each subsequent injection.

The intravenous anaesthetic agents of practical importance are thiopentone, thioamylal, and methohexitone. The two thiobarbiturates are about equally potent and do not differ clinically.

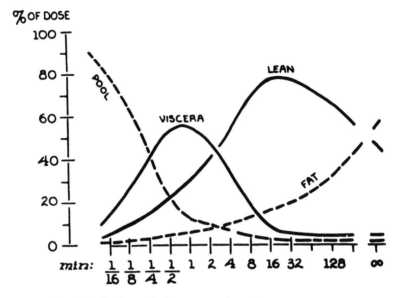

FIGURE 2 Distribution of thiopentone in different body tissues and organs at various times after its intravenous injection. From Price, et al. Clinical Pharmacology and Therapeutics. 1:16 (1960). C.V. Mosby, St. Louis, Mo.

Methohexitone is shorter acting and has a higher potency. These barbiturates in the form of their sodium salts are soluble, resulting in solutions that are highly alkaline (pH greater than 10.0) and are not stable over long periods. The solution should therefore be freshly prepared from the powder by adding distilled water and should not stand longer than a few days. The thiobarbiturates are used in a 2.5 per cent solution and the average dose is 5 mg per kilogram body weight in a healthy patient.

Clinically, barbiturates induce sleep rapidly but they block afferent impulses poorly (i.e. they have little analgesic effect) and provide almost no muscle relaxation. The central depression with intact afferent impulse activity may be the reason for the frequent occurrence of hyperactive reflex responses such as coughing or laryngospasm in response to minor stimulation.

Depression of respiration is directly related to the depth of anaesthesia. In deeper levels of anaesthesia the response to carbon dioxide is suppressed. Pharyngeal and glottic reflexes are also depressed, so that airway obstruction may occur if the jaw is not lifted forward and an airway inserted. Certainly the patient who cannot open his mouth or move his neck should not be given an ultra-short-acting barbiturate.

The intravenous injection of barbiturate may cause a fall in blood pressure, presumably due to suppression of peripheral vascular tone and myocardial depression. Great care must be exercised when the patient has a fixed cardiac output as occurs in hypovolaemia, cardiac failure, or cardiac valvular disease. The onset of action is delayed in patients with prolonged circulation time as in heart failure, and the inexperienced anaesthetist may mistake this for high tolerance.

Because of the lack of analgesia and muscle relaxation and the short duration of action, these drugs are used in combination with nitrous oxide, narcotics or other inhalation agents. Muscle relaxants are required for thoracic or abdominal operations. The return of consciousness is rapid and not usually associated with unpleasant reactions such as nausea and vomiting or confusion. The effects may persist, however, for several hours and during this time the patient must be protected from possible hazards such as driving a car or walking on the street. Occasionally patients recovering from thiopentone may exhibit shivering, irregular breathing, and peripheral cyanosis. This may be related to heat loss resulting from cutaneous vasodilatation and associated depression of central heat-regulating mechanisms.

These agents should be injected very slowly with constant observation of the patient's responses. The injection of a test dose of 2 to 5 cc allows an assessment of the response. In cases where rapid induction is required because of a full stomach and danger of aspiration, a minimal sleep dose should be given very quickly. This dose will be less than the usual sleep dose.

If thiopentone is injected into an artery by mistake a marked vasospasm occurs with occlusion of the arterial supply of the arm. This may result in gangrene unless adequate measures for treatment are instituted (see chapter 12).

Narcotics such as morphine, meperidine, and anileridine are commonly used as intravenous anaesthetic agents. In this group one may also include 'Innovar,' which is a combination of fentanyl, a potent narcotic, and droperidol, a major tranquillizer, and which is used to produce a state commonly called neuroleptanaesthesia. In this state the patient is relatively pain free but rousable. These agents, including Innovar, are also used to provide added analgesia in association with nitrous oxide anaesthesia combined with the use of muscle relaxants. They are administered by intermittent intravenous injection in small doses or by a dilute continuous infusion as required by the patient's response to painful stimuli. Large doses may cause respiratory depression or cardiovascular collapse in a hypovolaemic patient. This may be dangerous because the effect is prolonged as compared with the duration of an inhalational agent. These agents are popular at this time because of some of the late side-effects of the inhalation agents in use at present, including possible hypersensitivity to halothane or the products of its metabolism and the toxic effects of methoxyflurane on the kidney.

Diazepam (Valium) Useful an an induction agent in patients with an unstable cardiovascular system. The slow injection of 10 to 40 mg of Valium intravenously will usually provide sleep in about three minutes without much change in the blood pressure or pulse. It is also useful in cardioversion for the treatment of cardiac arrythmias. In patients who are allergic to barbiturates such as thiopentone, this may be the induction agent of choice.

Ketamine hydrochloride A new non-barbiturate general anaesthetic. It can be administered intravenously in a dose of 2 mg per kg body weight or by the intramuscular route in doses of 6 to 10 mg per kg body weight. It produces a state called 'dissociative anaesthesia,' which is characterized by good analgesia, retention of pharyngeal and glottic reflexes, minimal respiratory depression, increased blood pressure and pulse rate, and an increase in intracranial pressure. It does not block visceral pain pathways or provide suitable muscle relaxation, so that its indications are specific for procedures not requiring these features. Its use may be followed by unpleasant dreams or hallucination in adults and this limits its usefulness in patients over 12 years of age. Recovery time may be quite prolonged, so that it may not find acceptance for paediatric out-patient surgery. Its main indications seem to be for operations on the skin and musculoskeletal system, such as skin grafting or reduction of simple fractures. It is very useful when an airway may be difficult to obtain such as in the case of a burn contracture of the neck, because reflexes are retained.

METHODS OF ADMINISTRATION

The inhalation anaesthetic agents (gases and vapours) must be administered to the patient in known concentrations which are altered either to increase or to decrease the depth of anaesthesia. To achieve this control the anaesthetist uses an anaesthetic gas machine designed to produce known anaesthetic mixtures, which are then conveyed to the patient through a breathing circuit. The use of a breathing circuit assists the anaesthetist in monitoring tidal volume and respiratory rate as well as in allowing him to assist or control ventilation.

THE ANAESTHETIC MACHINE

The basic components of an anaesthetic machine are important because any defect can result in serious complications due to hypoxia, hypercarbia, or inaccurate dosage of inhalation anaesthetic agents. The basic components include compressed gases, pressure gauges, reducing valves, flow meters, vaporizers, and finally the breathing attachment.

Compressed Gases
The compressed gases (oxygen, nitrous oxide) are contained in cylinders attached to the anaesthetic machine. The oxygen tank contains gaseous oxygen at a pressure of about 2200 p.s.i. when full. Medical gas cylinders are colour coded. Oxygen cylinders have white neck and shoulders but are frequently entirely white; the nitrous oxide tank is similarly marked in blue and when full contains liquid nitrous oxide of a certain weight and gaseous nitrous oxide at a

pressure of 750 p.s.i. In many hospitals these cylinders are kept in reserve and the main gas supplies are piped into the operating room from a central storage bank of compressed gases in the hospital. Cyclopropane is also packed in a pressure cylinder and attached to the gas machine. It is an orange or chrome cylinder and the pressure is 75 p.s.i. All cylinders attached to the machine and outlets for gas lines have a pin index system to ensure that the gas is not attached to the wrong inlet. As an example, this will prevent nitrous oxide cylinders from being attached to an oxygen inlet, which could be a lethal error.

Pressure Gauges and Reducing Valves

There is usually a pressure gauge indicating the pressure in the cylinder at the point of entry of the gas. In the case of oxygen this will indicate how full the tank is. Tanks should not be used when the pressure is below 200 p.s.i. because of the dangerous consequences should an oxygen tank run out during the anaesthetic. Some anaesthetic machines have an alarm which indicates when an oxygen cylinder becomes empty, while others have a safety feature which turns off the nitrous oxide flow when the oxygen pressure falls to zero. The nitrous oxide pressure gauge shows decreasing gas pressure in the cylinder only when the liquid nitrous oxide has all been converted to the gaseous phase.

The high pressures of these gases within the storage cylinders must be reduced and held constant to permit measurement of gas flows by the flowmeters of the anaesthetic machine. This is accomplished by *reducing valves* placed in the line ahead of the flow meters.

Flow Meters

A flow meter is positioned downstream from the reducing valve to indicate the volume of gas flow during unit time. This is usually calibrated in litres per minute and must be accurate to ensure proper proportions of oxygen. Most machines use a modification of a variable orifice dry gas flow meter or a rotameter. The gas flows upward through a conical glass tube, raising a rotating ball or bobbin. As the bobbin rises the orifice through which the gas flows increases in diameter. The bobbin comes to rest where the pressure difference across the orifice is equal to the weight of the bobbin. Thus with proper calibration this will indicate the flow rate of the gas. Because viscosity (influencing laminar flow) and density (influencing flow through orifices) are specific and different for each gas, each flow meter must be calibrated for a particular gas.

After the gases pass through the flow meters they may proceed through vaporizers for volatile liquid agents prior to entering the breathing circuit.

Vaporizers

Vaporizers are required for the administration of volatile anaesthetic agents. In modern machines they are placed down stream from the flow meters so that a measured volume of gas from the flow meters may be passed constantly through the vaporizer.

The ether bottle on the Boyle type of anaesthetic machine is a simple type of vaporizer. By the opening of a valve the gas from the flow meter can be directed partially or totally through a glass jar partially filled with the volatile liquid anaesthetic. By adjustment of a second mechanism the gas may be directed either over the surface or bubbled through the liquid.

The vapour concentration thus obtained varies with the flow of gas and the temperature of the liquid. Evaporation uses heat and consequently the temperature of the liquid anaesthetic will fall; vapour pressure is in direct relation to the temperature of the liquid, and thus the output of vapour will decline with continued use. For this reason, the concentration of vapour produced by such a device is actually unknown, although its performance is predictable by experience and observation of the patient's response, and the anaesthetist will learn to operate the vaporizer safely.

Various vaporizers have been designed to achieve a predictable and measurable output of vapour. Ideally a vaporizer should yield an unchanging concentration of vapour at a given setting irrespective of variations of gas flow, liquid content, or temperature. At the present time two vaporizers which are widely used allow fairly accurate estimation of the vapour output.

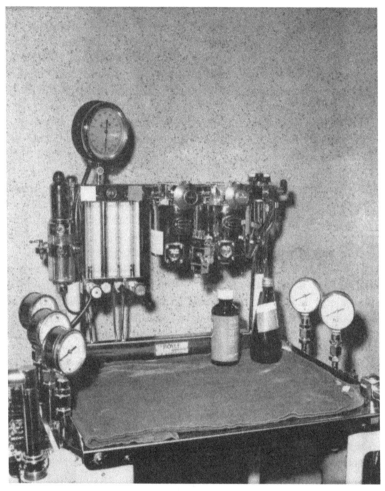

FIGURE 3   Top of anaesthetic machine showing pressure gauges, flow meters, and vaporizers

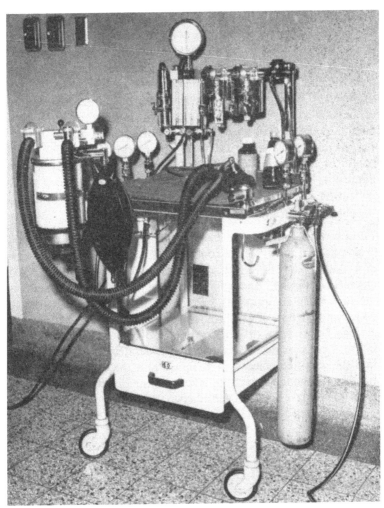

FIGURE 4   Anaesthetic machine showing circle breathing system with carbon dioxide absorber and nitrous oxide and oxygen cylinders attached

The copper kettle In the copper kettle vaporizer, the liquid is held in a copper container which is highly heat-conductive and so keeps temperature constant by transfer of heat from the room air and metal parts of the anaesthetic machine. A measured volume of oxygen from a separate flow meter is passed in a multitude of small bubbles through the liquid, producing saturated vapour at the temperature of the vaporizer. The known volume of a constant vapour is then diluted to the desired anaesthetic concentration by adding further oxygen or nitrous oxide. This type of vaporizer is used for ether, halothane, and methoxyflurane, and can be adapted for any volatile liquid anaesthetic. The concentration of vapour administered to the patient can be calculated from the dilution of the highly concentrated vapour coming from the vaporizer.

The Fluotec® vaporizer In the Fluotec® type vaporizer the liquid is also held in a conductive container. The total gas flow from the flow meter passes through the vaporizer, but only a portion of it is channelled through the vaporizing chamber. The temperature-sensitive valve compensates for temperature changes in the liquid by varying the flow of gas through the vapour chamber. The vaporizer can be set for a desired percentage of vapour (for halothane, 0.5 to 4 per cent) which is delivered accurately if the flow of gas into the vaporizer exceeds 4 L/min. From the vaporizer the prepared anaesthetic gas mixture is fed into the breathing circuit. This type of vaporizer has also been adapted for methoxyflurane (Pentec) and may be specifically calibrated for any volatile liquid agent.

Breathing Attachments and Circuits

The prepared anaesthetic gas mixture can be conducted to the patient in a number of ways. However, any method used must take the following factors into consideration:

1 *Respiratory rate and tidal volume* of a patient vary over a wide range. Regardless of such variations there must be an adequate volume of gas available in the breathing system at any time for each breath, regardless of its volume. This can be accomplished with a reservoir bag (usually a rubber bag) with a volume of 1 to 5 litres

depending on the range of tidal volume possible. While the gas machine delivers a continuous flow of gas into the reservoir bag the patient can inspire intermittently out of the reservoir.

2 *Resistance* All anaesthetic systems must allow unobstructed breathing. This makes it mandatory for conducting tubes and connections interposed between the patient and the reservoir bag to be of sufficient diameter to offer no resistance, within the range of flow rates of inspiration and expiration. All valves in the system must function at the lowest possible opening pressure. Children may be anaesthetized using a circuit (Ayre's T-piece with reservoir) without an expiratory blow-off valve to minimize resistance to exhalation. Flexible tubes must be corrugated to avoid kinking.

3 *Carbon dioxide removal* Anaesthetic breathing systems must be designed to allow effective elimination of carbon dioxide. This can be accomplished either by a flow of gases sufficient to prevent rebreathing or by the use of a carbon dioxide absorption system. A CO_2 absorber must remove carbon dioxide efficiently over a long period of time and have no appreciable resistance to air flow. It cannot be used with trichlorethylene administration because of the formation of toxic products.

Breathing circuits are usually attached to the anaesthetic machine by an adjustable bracket and a connecting tube for the fresh gas inflow. Machines differ in this regard so that some machines have a simple tube which may be attached to different breathing circuits while others (Boyle's machine) may have a modified switch which directs the gases to either the semi-open or the closed circuit. All circuits have connectors for either a face mask or tracheal tube, a conducting tube or tubes, which are corrugated to avoid kinking, and a reservoir bag. Other parts of the circuits will be discussed below. The basic choice of circuits may be divided into semi-open, closed, or semi-closed systems.

Semi-Open
This system allows the exhaled gas to pass into the external atmo-

sphere. There may be some degree of rebreathing. This is determined by the volume of flow of fresh gas and can be eliminated if the flow is large enough. There is a single corrugated breathing tube in this system.

The Magill Attachment

This attachment was described by Sir Ivan Magill, an eminent British anaesthetist. It consists of a reservoir bag at the gas machine, a conducting tube, and an expiratory blow-off valve at the mask or tracheal tube (Fig. 5). During expiration the reservoir bag is filled by the continuous gas flow and the patient's expiration. With the proper flow rate (equals patient's minute volume) the reservoir bag is filled during the early part of expiration and the pressure rises

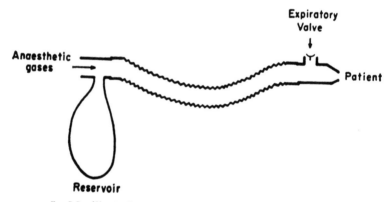

FIGURE 5   Magill attachment

sufficiently to open the expiratory valve. The second portion of the expired gas, including the alveolar air with a high CO_2 concentration, is then blown off to the atmosphere. This system is useful during spontaneous respiration but should not be used when controlled ventilation is instituted, as the compression of the breathing bag with the partially closed blow-off valve will cause the patient to rebreathe CO_2. It is used with agents that cannot be used with the CO_2 absorber, such as trichloroethylene. It should not be used for very small children owing to the resistance of the expiratory blow-off valve.

The Ayre's T-Piece System

Ayre's T is essentially a non-rebreathing system, if an adequate fresh gas inflow is used. The anaesthetic mixture is directed into the T at the attachment of the mask or the endotracheal tube. The patient's expiration and fresh gas will escape through the open-end of the T which is attached to a corrugated tube. A small breathing bag with an open end is attached to this corrugated tube in the Jackson-Rees modification. The opening in the tail of the bag is adjusted to permit gas to escape without resistance (Fig. 6). This is a simple technique; the equipment is light and requires no valves. Assisted ventila-

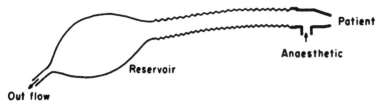

FIGURE 6 Ayre's T-piece with reservoir

tion may be accomplished by intermittently closing the vent at the end of the reservoir bag with the thumb and the first finger. It may be difficult to use this circuit in adults because of the high gas flow required. A respirator can be attached instead of the reservoir bag, to facilitate controlled ventilation.

Non-Rebreathing System

If a non-rebreathing or one-way valve (Fig. 7) is interposed at the face mask or the tracheal tube in the Magill circuit previously described, a 'non-rebreathing' circuit is formed. The patient inhales the anaesthetic gas from the reservoir bag and exhales the gas directly into the room. The valves commonly used for this purpose are the Reuben valve and the Stephen-Slater valve. The valve must be as close as possible to the patient's airway since the volume of the anaesthetic equipment between the airway and the valve represents mechanical dead-space. This system requires a fresh gas inflow at least equal to the minute volume of the patient.

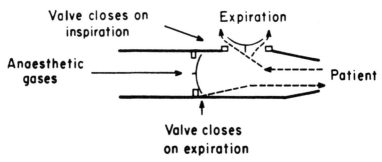

FIGURE 7 Non-breathing valve

BREATHING SYSTEMS WITH CO_2 ABSORPTION

Anaesthetic breathing circuits may include a carbon dioxide absorber. Such systems may be used either in a closed mode, or by a semi-closed technique. In the closed system there is total rebreathing of expired gas from which the CO_2 is absorbed. The only additions which need be made consist of metabolic requirements of oxygen, and the anaesthetic agent absorbed by the tissues and required for the induction and maintenance of an appropriate plane of anaesthesia. Oxygen consumption will vary from 200 to 300 cc per minute in the adult, and there will be some mechanical loss from most anaesthetic circuits. Sufficient oxygen must be added to ensure that an adequate concentration of oxygen is available in the inspired gas. It must also be remembered that as these gases are rebreathed, the concentration of the inhalation anaesthetic agent may be less than that delivered from the vaporizer, and appropriate increments of the anaesthetic agent must be added to the circuit to maintain the desired level of anaesthesia. Manually controlled ventilation can be instituted effectively with the closed system, or a mechanical ventilator may be attached in place of the reservoir bag.

Closed breathing systems may be of the To-and-Fro or Circle type.

To-and-Fro Technique

The 'To and Fro' closed breathing system consists essentially of a chimney piece incorporating a spring-loaded blow-off valve and a gas inlet, adapted at the patient end to fit a face mask or tracheal tube, and leading, at the other extremity, to a reservoir bag, with CO_2 absorption canister interposed between. This system has the disadvantages that very bulky equipment must be supported in the region of the patient's face, and it is very rarely used today.

Circle Breathing System

The circle breathing system incorporates two breathing tubes, one leading the inspired gas to the patient, and the other conducting expired gas away from the patient. Gas flow in this system is directed

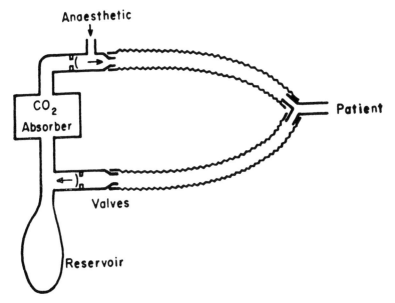

FIGURE 8   Circle breathing system

in a circle by two directional valves. The system also incorporates a reservoir bag, a CO_2 absorber, a gas inlet which is usually on the inspiratory side of the circuit, and a blow-off valve in which the tension may be regulated by a spring and screw arrangement (Fig. 8).

Semi-Closed Technique

When a flow larger than the gas and vapour being metabolized or absorbed by the body is introduced into the closed system, the excess gas must be vented to the outside air to prevent inappropriate increase of pressure. This venting is achieved by adjustment of the blow-off valve provided in the closed system. Small flows of gas may be used, provided the proper concentrations are achieved. It must be remembered that with small flows the metabolic consumption of oxygen may reduce the oxygen available in the inspired gas, and the flow rates must be adequate to prevent this. For example, if the inflow of oxygen is reduced much below 1000 cc per minute in a nitrous oxide–oxygen mixture, gradual reduction of oxygen concentration in the breathing system will occur. It must also be remembered that concentration of a volatile anaesthetic agent may be less in the inspired mixture than that delivered from the vaporizer.

Manually controlled ventilation can be instituted effectively with the semi-closed system if there is meticulous regulation of the blow-off valve. A mechanical ventilator can likewise be attached in place of the reservoir bag, as with the closed system. It is easier to maintain steady concentrations of the components of the anaesthetic mixture with the semi-closed system and moderate flows of gas than it is with the completely closed circuit. On the other hand, the closed circuit has a distinct advantage in circumstances where explosive or inflammable agents are used, since it avoids the venting of these dangerous substances into the atmosphere.

PROBLEMS WITH BREATHING CIRCUITS

The rubber corrugated tubing in breathing circuits dissolves halothane or methoxyflurane in fairly large amounts. Therefore even when other anaesthetics are administered, a patient may inhale significant amounts of these agents when the tubing has been used in a previous case. To prevent this the tubing must be vented for a considerable period of time and this becomes impractical in many situations.

The breathing circuit becomes very moist due to condensation of the exhaled water vapour and bacteria may flourish. Therefore, a system must be developed by which these breathing circuits can be sterilized to prevent the transmission of infection from patient to patient. This may be an indication for the use of disposable anaesthetic circuits.

The inhalation anaesthetic agents that are exhaled into the room from the blow-off valve may, over long periods of time, be injurious to the operating room personnel. Significant levels of halothane and methoxyflurane have been found in the operating rooms in proximity to the anaesthetist, the surgeons, and the nurses. From what is known of the effects of halothane on the immune response, this may be harmful over a long period. Therefore, methods for removing these gases from the operating room must be employed. These include various suction attachments to the expiratory valve to draw the gases out of the operating room. Adequate operating room ventilation is also a necessity.

Very high pressures can be built up in some breathing circuits if the blow-off valve is closed by mistake and the fresh gas inflow is continued. These high pressures in the circuit and in the patient's airway can result in tension pneumothorax or subcutaneous emphysema. Therefore, these breathing circuits should be equipped with pressure-limiting valves to protect patients from these complications of excessive airway pressure.

CARBON DIOXIDE ABSORPTION

In carbon dioxide absorption systems, carbon dioxide is brought into contact with water, forming carbonic acid which is then neutralized through combination with a base. The bases usually employed are the hydroxides of sodium, calcium, or barium; of these sodium hydroxide has the greatest activity.

Commercial soda lime consists of 5 per cent $NaOH$ and 95 per cent $Ca(OH)_2$. These agents are compressed either in pellets or granules. To achieve greater hardness, silica is added. The granules must be of sufficient size to allow the free flow of air between them, and they must not crumble or form dust.

The chemical reactions which take place in the absorption of carbon dioxide can be represented by the following equations:

$$CO_2 + H_2O \rightarrow H_2CO_3,$$
$$H_2CO_3 + 2NaOH \rightarrow Na_2CO_3 + 2H_2O \text{ (rapid reaction)},$$
$$H_2CO_3 + Ca(OH)_2 \rightarrow CaCO_3 + 2H_2O \text{ (slow reaction)},$$

also

$$Na_2CO_3 + Ca(OH)_2 \rightarrow CaCO_3 + 2NaOH \text{ (regeneration)}.$$

During these reactions heat is liberated and soda lime canisters will become warm as carbon dioxide is absorbed. A colour indicator is usually added to the soda lime to indicate when the absorbing capacity has been exhausted.

INHALATION TECHNIQUES WITHOUT A GAS MACHINE

Inhalation anaesthesia can be administered in situations where an anaesthetic machine is not available. The oldest method was by the open drop technique. A mask covered with eight or more layers of gauze is placed over the patient's mouth and nose and a volatile liquid anaesthetic (ether, vinethene, ethyl chloride, chloroform) is dropped onto the gauze from a bottle with a suitable dropper. The air stream of the patient's respiration vaporizes the liquid and the patient inhales a mixture of anaesthetic vapour and air. This technique is used very little at present in Canadian hospitals as it does not provide satisfactory conditions for most operations.

Draw-over Vaporizers

Some vaporizers can be used without compressed gases. In recent examples room air is drawn through a suitably modified calibrated halothane vaporizer, and the E.M.O. machine is useful in situations where compressed gases are not available. The incorporation of a self-inflating reservoir bag (Ambu, pulmonator, etc.) can be useful to assist ventilation in these circumstances.

MANAGEMENT OF A GENERAL ANAESTHETIC

A safe and effective general anaesthetic requires careful preparation to avoid complications. The patient must be assessed preoperatively so that techniques, drugs and their dosages are appropriate. The needs of the surgical procedures are very relevant because some operations will require profound analgesia while others will need complete muscle paralysis. Finally, equipment and drugs must be available ready for any occurrence. Suction equipment must be checked; the anaesthetic circuits must be properly assembled so that the patient can be ventilated with oxygen, and equipment such as the laryngoscope, airway and tracheal tubes should be ready to secure an airway. Drugs that must be immediately available include a short-acting muscle relaxant (succinylcholine), and a vasopressor. An added useful precaution is the use of an indwelling needle in a vein so that drugs can be given quickly in an emergency situation.

Induction of anaesthesia in most patients is carried out by the use of a rapid acting intravenous agent such as thiopentone. This does not disturb the patient or produce excitement. This technique may not be suitable in patients with airway obstruction, shock, or lack of accessible veins. Sometimes a rapid acting non-irritating inhalation agent such as nitrous oxide followed by halothane is used for induction in children. The child can usually be talked into blowing up 'the balloon' (the reservoir bag). By continual talking in a quiet voice, the anaesthetist can usually induce the child with a minimum of struggle. For this inhalation induction it is necessary to use moderately high concentrations until a suitable alveolar tension of the agent is achieved. Following induction the concentration may be decreased to maintenance level. When halothane is used, this concentration is usually about 1 per cent whereas with methoxyflurane maintenance concentration varies between 0.5 and 0.8 per cent. At present the majority of techniques are based on the use of nitrous oxide as a vehicle or carrier gas. As a sole anaesthetic agent it is rarely suitable because of its low potency. The use of 50 to 70 per cent nitrous oxide with oxygen provides some loss of consciousness and analgesia. When this gas mixture is supplemented by other inhalation or intravenous agents the mixture provides more adequate surgical anaesthesia than could be achieved with the same doses of the supplementary agent alone. Since nitrous oxide has few side-effects compared with the undesirable effects of high doses of potent inhalation agents, such balanced anaesthesia has fewer drug-induced complications than anaesthesia produced by the use of one potent agent alone. This mixture is suitable to vaporize volatile anaesthetics and it provides analgesic properties in combination with agents such as halothane that in themselves may have minimal analgesic effects.

Because of its solubility, nitrous oxide comes out of solution in the blood very quickly, when the concentration in the inspired gas is reduced at the end of operation. Nitrous oxide then diffuses rapidly into the lungs, diluting the oxygen present in the alveoli. It is wise, therefore, to administer 100 per cent oxygen for three minutes at the end of operation to avoid the effects of this diffusion hypoxia.

During anaesthesia it is necessary to maintain an accurate anaesthetic record. This includes a graph on which blood pressure, pulse, respiratory rate, temperature, and central venous pressure may be continuously recorded and on which changes may be seen easily and quickly. Doses and the time of administration of drugs must be included in this record so that their effects and the duration of action can be considered. Any complications should be recorded so that a future anaesthetist will be warned in advance to take certain precautions.

At the end of anaesthesia in the operating room the patient is transferred to a recovery room by the anaesthetist, where specially trained nurses continue the care of this often unconscious patient. The anaesthetist's responsibility continues in this area, at least until the patient is fully awake and his protective reflexes have returned. Any patient whose state is unstable in any way will require the close supervision of the anaesthetist for as long as necessary. It is also advisable that the anaesthetist visit the patient on the following day to ensure that no complications have arisen that could be related to the anaesthetic management.

REFERENCES

DRIPPS, R.D.; ECKENHOFF, J.E. & VANDAM, L.D. Introduction to Anesthesia. Philadelphia & London: W.B. Saunders Company.

WYLIE, W.D. & CHURCHILL-DAVIDSON, H.C. A Practice of Anaesthesia (1972). Chicago: Year Book Medical Publishers.

GRAY, T.C. & NUNN, J.F. General Anaesthesia (1971). London: Butterworth.

JONE CHANG

5

Neuromuscular transmission and muscle relaxation

The history of muscle relaxants has its known origin in the sixteenth century. In 1595 Sir Walter Raleigh published his *Discovery of Guiana* which first mentioned that the South American Indians used a poisoned arrow that actually contained crude curare. The work of Claude Bernard in 1850 showed that injection of curare into the frog paralysed the animal without alteration of nerve conduction or muscle irritability in response to direct stimulation.

Curare was first used in anaesthesia in 1942 by Griffith and Johnson in Montreal. The introduction of this relaxant drug into clinical anaesthesia has brought a new era in the development and advancement of safer anaesthesia.

PHYSIOLOGY OF NEUROMUSCULAR TRANSMISSION

Motor nerve fibres end in the muscle to form synapses. These sites are known as the 'neuromuscular junctions,' the 'myoneural junctions,' or the 'motor end plates.' The neuromuscular junction consists of a presynaptic membrane and a postsynaptic membrane. The presynaptic and postsynaptic membranes are separated by an intervening space, the synaptic cleft, which represents a real discontinuity between the nerve and muscle. The interior of the postsynaptic membrane has high potassium and low sodium content. This unequal distribution of electrolytes creates a potention difference of −90 millivolts, known as the resting end-plate potential.

When an impulse from the motor nerve reaches the neuromuscular junction, acetylcholine is liberated from the area of the presynaptic membrane. The acetylcholine crosses the synaptic cleft and produces a change in permeability of the postsynaptic membrane. The increased permeability causes an outflow of potassium from the interior of the postsynaptic membrane and an inflow of sodium. With the equalization of electrolytes, the resting potential is diminished to zero millivolts. At this point the membrane is completely depolarized. The depolarization initiates potential changes and depolarization of the adjacent muscle fibre, resulting in contraction of the muscle.

The acetylcholine released at the neuromuscular junction is soon hydrolysed to acetic acid and choline by the action of acetylcholinesterase. The permeability of the membrane returns to the normal resting state and the electrolytes are restored actively to the previous unequal distribution, i.e. high potassium and low sodium. When the electrolyte concentrations again show the marked gradient, the membrane is repolarized.

NEUROMUSCULAR BLOCK

Neuromuscular block is an interference with the transmission of the nerve impulse through the neuromuscular junction to the muscle fibres with resulting relaxation of the affected muscle fibres. In normal neuromuscular transmission, depolarization and repolarization occur at the neuromuscular junction; thus interference with the normal response at any stage will result in neuromuscular blockade. There are two groups of drugs available for the production of neuromuscular blockade: one interferes with the depolarization of the membrane, the other interferes with its repolarization. The neuromuscular blocking agents are therefore divided into two main groups, the non-depolarizing or competitive blockers and the depolarizing blockers.

Non-Depolarizing (Competitive) Blockers
Non-depolarizing or competitive blocking agents are usually quater-

nary ammonium compounds which resemble the structure of acetylcholine but do not mimic its action. The compounds compete with acetylcholine at the receptor site so that the released acetylcholine does not produce changes in the postsynaptic membrane. In other words the non-depolarizing blocking agents, by producing a stable membrane, prevent the acetylcholine from depolarizing the membrane or end plate. Thus the muscle loses tone and relaxes. If greater amounts of acetylcholine or similar substances are present the acetylcholine can displace the blocking agent and produce depolarization of the membrane. Clinically, neostigmine increases the concentration of acetylcholine by destroying cholinesterase and preventing the hydrolysis of acetylcholine, thus counteracting the non-depolarizing neuromuscular blockers.

The characteristic features of the non-depolarizing neuromuscular block are: (*a*) Potential fades with stimulation of the nerve, whether by a single impulse or by tetany, or the muscle power fades with nerve stimulation. (*b*) Post-tetanic facilitation is present. (*c*) Fade and post-tetanic facilitation are removed with neostigmine (Fig. 1).

When the nerve is stimulated by tetanic or single electrical impulses, the evoked potential or muscle power gradually decreases in the muscles blocked by non-depolarizing blockers. If immediately after a tetanic stimulation the nerve is again stimulated, the potential or muscle power is improved temporarily. This phenomenon, known as facilitation, is due to the persistence of acetylcholine at the neuromuscular junction following the tetany, which reinforces the acetylcholine released by subsequent nerve stimulation. Finally, when neostigmine is given, the response at the neuromuscular junction is restored to normal because the acetylcholine-esterase is inhibited by neostigmine, so that the duration of acetylcholine action is increased.

Depolarizing Neuromuscular Blockers

Depolarizing blocking agents are compounds which resemble acetylcholine in structure and action. They act by increasing the permeability of the postsynaptic membrane, thus initiating depolarization. Since these agents are slowly broken down, the increased permeability of the membrane is maintained and the potassium–

Non-depolarizing Block   Depolarizing Block

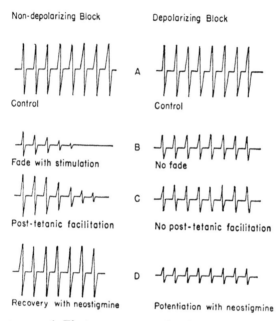

FIGURE 1 Electromyograms showing typical responses to the two types of muscle relaxant

sodium ratio is not restored to normal after depolarization; thus there is no repolarization. When the membrane is maintained in this state no further response can be initiated. This produces neuromuscular block to nerve stimulation.

The characteristic features of depolarizing block are: (*a*) Potential or muscle power does not fade with stimulation of the nerve. (*b*) Post-tetanic facilitation is absent. (*c*) Fade occurs with neostigmine (Fig. 1).

When the nerve is stimulated, the evoked potential is depressed by the depolarization block but the depressed potential and the muscle power remain constant. If, after tetanic stimulation, the nerve is stimulated with single twitches, the potential is not altered, i.e., there is no post-tetanic facilitation. When depolarizing block is present, neostigmine will increase it, so that stimulation of the nerve will produce smaller potential and weaker muscle response.

Neostigmine increases the duration of acetylcholine action, thus potentiating the depolarizing blockers. The respective actions of depolarizing and non-depolarizing blockers are shown in Figure 1.

Dual Block
The term dual block is used in connection with an initial depolarizing block which, in time, converts into a non-depolarizing block. Dual block occurs only with the depolarizing relaxants. If large doses of depolarizing agents are administered over a period of time, there is a gradual transformation in the responses of the postsynaptic membrane as the type of block shifts from a pure depolarizing block to a pure non-depolarizing (competitive) one. During the intervening period there is a combination of depolarizing and non-depolarizing blocks, giving a bizarre picture of response to stimulation and to neostigmine. Once the change is complete, the response of the membrane is similar to that associated with non-depolarizing blockers.

Competitive (Non-Depolarizing) and Non-Competitive (Depolarizing) Block
Feldman recently advanced a new theory to supplant the theory of competition for the non-depolarizing blockers. This theory postulates that competitive or non-depolarizing blockers do not compete with the ACH at the receptor sites but form a stable receptor complex which prevents access of ACH to the receptor sites. The displacement of these receptor-complexes are dependent upon the total quanta of ACH rather than the plasma concentration. Large or prolonged dosage of depolarizing blockers may form loose receptor-complexes which are similar in action to the non-depolarizing blockers. This action explains the formation of phase I to phase II block, i.e. dual block.

Neostigmine and Edrophonium
Neostigmine and edrophonium are classified as anticholinesterase drugs. Basically they inhibit the action of acetylcholinesterase, the enzyme that catalyses the degradation of acetylcholine to acetic acid and choline. Thus, anticholinesterase prolongs the action of acetyl-

choline. In addition, both neostigmine and edrophonium are themselves depolarizing agents, i.e., they directly depolarize the postsynaptic membrane. The combination of actions counteracts the non-depolarizing (competitive) blockers and potentiates the blocking activity of the depolarizing blockers.

Neostigmine, with greater anticholinesterase activity, is effective for a longer time. Edrophonium is mainly a depolarizer and has a fleeting duration of action – less than five minutes.

MUSCLE RELAXATION

The desired result of neuromuscular blockade is muscle relaxation, which is very important in facilitating certain types of surgery. The advent of muscle relaxants greatly increased the safety of anaesthesia. Prior to their use, relaxation of muscles for operation was obtained with deep general anaesthesia. Since deep anaesthesia is depressing to a wide variety of homeostatic and metabolic functions, long operations were very poorly tolerated, especially by poor-risk patients. When muscle relaxants are employed to obtain adequate muscle relaxation, only light general anaesthesia is required, and depression is consequently minimal. As a result, long surgical operations are well tolerated by both good-risk and poor-risk patients.

Those muscle relaxants which are useful clinically are divided into two groups: the non-depolarizing or competitive group including d-tubocurarine, gallamine, and a new non-depolarizing blocker, pancuronium; and the depolarizing group with decamethonium and succinylcholine.

D-Tubocurarine, Gallamine and Pancuronium

D-tubocurarine, a purified alkaloid of natural curare, is a non-depolarizing type of muscle-relaxant drug. It has a long duration of action. Depending on the dose, the effect may last from thirty to forty-five minutes. When d-tubocurarine is administered slowly extraocular muscles are the first to be affected, followed by the muscles of the head and neck, the periphery, and finally the muscles of respiration. The diaphragm and the accessory muscles of respiration are the last to be paralysed. During recovery from neuro-muscular blockade, muscle function returns in the reverse order. When adequate relaxation is obtained, all striated muscles are partially or completely paralysed, including the muscles of respiration. Therefore the most important prerequisite for clinical adminis-tration of d-tubocurarine and other muscle relaxants is that ade-quate ventilation be maintained at all times.

The action of d-tubocurarine is synergistic with diethyl ether, and thus a smaller dose of d-tubocurarine is required with ether anaesthesia. D-tubocurarine relaxation may be reversed with neo-stigmine. Edrophonium (Tensilon), because of its very brief action, is useful only as a testing agent for reversing d-tubocurarine and non-depolarizing blockers.

Gallamine (Flaxedil®) and Pancuronium are synthetic quater-nary ammonium compounds. The clinical response at the neuro-muscular junction is exactly the same as with d-tubocurarine.

Autonomic nervous system Autonomic ganglia are blocked by d-tubocurarine in large doses. This may precipitate hypotension in hypovolaemic patients or in those with fixed cardiac output. Gallamine blocks the cardiac depressor nerves so that sinus tachy-cardia of greater or lesser degree may result. Heart rates as rapid as 150 beats per minute are occasionally encountered.

Cardiovascular system D-tubocurarine may produce hypotension. Gallamine tachycardia is fairly common. Pancuronium does not alter the blood pressure or heart rate.

Respiratory system The influence of d-tubocurarine, pancuronium, and gallamine on the respiratory system is indirect. When the muscles of respiration are paralysed by the relaxant drugs, complete apnoea or inadequate ventilation is the result. D-tubocurarine may induce histamine release and produce bronchospasm.

Central nervous system Under usual anaesthetic conditions d-tubo-curarine, pancuronium, and gallamine have no known effect on the central nervous system. Only under abnormal conditions of pro-longed apnoea do the relaxant drugs have an influence. As long as the state of apnoea is present the patient remains unconscious. Once spontaneous respiration is initiated the patient becomes conscious. At present it is not known whether the afferent or central mechanism is depressed.

Histamine release D-tubocurarine is capable of causing histamine release which may result in bronchoconstriction or hypotension. This effect is very minor with pancuronium and gallamine. Histamine release resulting in clinical difficulties is uncommon.

Metabolism D-tubocurarine is partly inactivated by conjugation in the liver and is partly excreted by the kidneys. Gallamine is entirely excreted by the kidneys. Pancuronium is mainly excreted by the kidneys.

Dose The average adult dose of d-tubocurarine is 15 to 30 mg, of pancuronium 2 to 5 mg, and of gallamine 100 to 200 mg, depending on the size and age of the patient. When ether is the main anaesthetic agent, the amount is reduced to between one-half and one-third of the initial dose because ether is synergistic with the non-depolarizing blockers.

Decamethonium and Succinylcholine

Both decamethonium and succinylcholine are synthetic depolarizing relaxant drugs. Decamethonium is longer acting, with a duration of action approximately 15 to 20 minutes, while succinylcholine is shorter acting, with a duration of 2 to 5 minutes. Initially the depolarizing blockers produce fasciculation of the muscles. This is usually seen with succinylcholine but only occasionally with decamethonium. The muscles are relaxed in the same sequence as with the non-depolarizers. Large doses of either decamethonium or succinylcholine will lead to a dual block response and potential prolonged apnoea. If the dual block response is complete, i.e., if the block has changed from the depolarizing to a non-depolarizing block, the blockade may be reversed by neostigmine or edrophonium. If the block is still in the depolarizing phase, no agents known at present will reverse it. Neostigmine administered during the depolarizing phase enhances the blockade.

Cardiovascular system Decamethonium has no effect on the cardiovascular system. Succinylcholine, on the other hand, not un-commonly produces bradycardia, especially in children. The brady-cardia may be prevented or corrected by adequate doses of atropine.

Respiratory system Both decamethonium and succinylcholine in-fluence the respiratory system indirectly by paralysis of the respira-tory muscles.

Central nervous system The responses of the central nervous system to decamethonium and succinylcholine are similar to those en-countered with the non-depolarizers.

Metabolism Decamethonium is excreted unchanged by the kidneys. Succinylcholine is degraded by circulating plasma cholinesterases to succinyl-monocholine and finally to choline and succinic acid. Some individuals exhibit an inherited plasma cholinesterase abnormality. This atypical plasma cholinesterase does not catalyse the decom-position of succinylcholine, and in such patients succinylcholine will have a prolonged action, resulting in prolonged apnoea. Atypical plasma cholinesterase may be detected by the dibucaine test devised by Kalow.

Dose The clinical dose of decamethonium is 3 to 5 mg. This dose should not be repeated. The initial dose of succinylcholine may vary from 20 to 100 mg. Subsequently any dose may be repeated or a continous intravenous drip may be used to maintain muscle relaxation.

Clinical application (*a*) Muscle relaxation for surgical operations. (*b*) For tracheal intubation. (*c*) To facilitate controlled respiration during anaesthesia. (*d*) To facilitate prolonged controlled ventila-tion in cases of respiratory insufficiency or other respiratory diffi-culties. (*e*) To modify electroconvulsive therapy. (*f*) To reduce muscle spasm. (*g*) To diagnose myasthenia gravis.

Choice of Relaxant Drugs
When prolonged relaxation is required, as for laparotomy or pro-longed ventilation, the longer acting non-depolarizing drugs such as d-tubocurarine, pancuronium, and gallamine are useful. The

doses may be repeated and the blockade can be reversed by neo-stigmine at the end of the operation. Decamethonium should not be used for long procedures because repeated doses will lead to dual block and possible prolonged apnoea.

When only a brief duration of relaxation is required, as for intubation or electroconvulsive therapy, succinylcholine is the agent of choice.

D-tubocurarine is useful in the diagnosis of myasthenia gravis because myasthenic patients are very sensitive to d-tubocurarine and gallamine.

Decamethonium test for diagnosis of myasthenia gravis is very useful and most diagnostic.

Complications

The most important complication of any type of neuromuscular blockade is prolonged action resulting in prolonged apnoea. In the non-depolarizing group, hypersensitivity associated with myasthenia gravis, severe electrolyte imbalance, or acidosis may lead to pro-longed apnoea and resistance to neostigmine reversal.

With the depolarizing group, large doses may result in dual block response and prolonged apnoea. With succinylcholine, prolonged apnoea is encountered most commonly in patients with atypical pseudocholinesterase, and rarely in those with low pseudocholin-esterase levels.

The primary treatment of prolonged apnoea is the maintenance of respiration until muscle power recovers. Usually the patient re-mains unconscious for the duration of the apnoea.

Succinylcholine may increase serum potassium level to an extent capable of producing cardiac asystole in severe burns, severe trauma, and neurological disorders such as spinal cord injuries and motor neurone disease. Finally succinylcholine may trigger the onset of malignant hyperthermia. This is frequently preceded by increase in muscle tone with the administration of succinylcholine.

Other complications are of minor importance.

6
Regional anaesthesia

Abolition of painful impulses from any part or parts of the body by temporarily interrupting the conductivity of sensory nerves with local anaesthetics is termed 'regional anaesthesia.' Motor function may or may not be affected, and the patient does not lose consciousness.

The broad term 'regional anaesthesia' may be subdivided into:

1 *Local application* ('topical') analgesic ointment and analgesic aerosol.

2 *Local infiltration* direct infiltration of an anaesthetic solution into the skin, wound, or lesion.

3 *Nerve block* direct infiltration of an anaesthetic solution into or around a peripheral nerve, or a group of peripheral nerves, e.g. the sciatic nerve, brachial plexus.

4 *Spinal or subarachnoid block* direct injection of a local anaesthetic solution into the subarachnoid space.

5 *Epidural or peridural block* direct injection of a local anaesthetic solution into the epidural or peridural space within the vertebral canal.

ANATOMY AND PHYSIOLOGY OF A PERIPHERAL NERVE

To understand how a local anaesthetic acts, one should refresh his basic knowledge of a peripheral nerve. A mixed peripheral nerve is composed of numerous individual fibres. Some may be covered with myelin, hence the classification into myelinated and non-myelinated fibres. A peripheral sensory fibre is the axon of a nerve cell, the body of which is located in a dorsal root ganglion. The cell body of the motor fibre is situated in the ventral horn of the spinal cord. Sensory fibres carry messages from the periphery, i.e., the skin, muscles, and joints, while motor fibres transmit messages to the muscles. Sensory fibres and motor fibres lie side by side in a peripheral nerve, and therefore both may be exposed simultaneously to the action of a local anaesthetic solution applied to the nerve.

NERVE BLOCK

Any peripheral nerve or group of peripheral nerves may be anaesthetized or blocked by a local anaesthetic solution, providing they are readily accessible by needle. A thorough knowledge of the anatomy involved is essential.

The more popular nerve blocks employed are for anaesthesia of: (*a*) *Upper Extremity* – Brachial Plexus Block via the Axillary or Supraclavicular approach. The former approach is recommended, as it eliminates the possibility of a pneumothorax, a complication of the supra-clavicular approach. (*b*) *Hand* – Median, ulnar, and radial nerve block at the wrist level. (*c*) *Upper Abdomen* – Bilateral intercostal nerve block plus splanchnic nerve block for intra-abdominal procedures. (*d*) *Lower Extremity* – Sciatic and Femoral Nerve Block. (*e*) *Intravenous Regional Anaesthesia* is an excellent technique to produce anaesthesia of the upper extremity.

The specific techniques for the various blocks will not be outlined in this precis. They may be studied in detail in any textbook on regional anaesthesia.

The modern local anaesthetic solutions recommended are lidocaine (Xylocaine) 0.5 to 2 per cent; propitocaine (Citanest) 1 to 3 per cent; mepivacaine (Carbocaine) 1 to 2 per cent; bupivacaine (Marcaine) 0.25 to 0.5 per cent. Tetracaine (Pontocaine) and procaine (Novocaine) are also used in some centres, but the first four drugs are preferable.

Reactions may occur when using local anaesthetic agents for nerve blocks. The operator must be familiar with the toxicity of the drugs employed, the reactions that may occur, and the proper methods of resuscitation.

SPINAL BLOCK

Spinal or subarachnoid block implies the direct injection of a local anaesthetic agent into the subarachnoid space. The usual site of injection is the interspace between the third and fourth lumbar vertebrae, although the interspaces 2–3, and 4–5 may be used. One should remember that the spinal cord in the adult usually terminates at the level of the body of the first lumbar vertebra, and any injection should be made below this level.

The spinal anaesthetic agents which are available today are safe. They are not neurotoxic in proper concentrations; they are packaged under sterile conditions and can be resterilized without loss of potency. These agents are dissolved in various diluents, e.g. saline, glucose solution, cerebrospinal fluid, or vasoconstrictors, allowing a wide choice of action and deposition.

The specific gravity of spinal fluid is 1.007. Spinal anaesthetic agents with various diluents added may be lighter than spinal fluid, and therefore termed *hypobaric*, or heavier than spinal fluid and termed *hyperbaric*. The *baricity* of the agent injected influences spread in the spinal fluid, and allows controllability of spread by posture.

The most popular local anaesthetic used for spinal anaesthesia today is tetracaine (Pontocaine); it is the only agent recommended for use by the part-time occasional anaesthetist. Some agents have lost their popularity, e.g. procaine (Novocaine), lidocaine (Xylocaine), and dibucaine (Nupercaine). Tetracaine is an ester of para-aminobenzoic acid and is similar in structure to procaine. Although it is seven to ten times as toxic as procaine, it is also ten times as potent, and can therefore be employed with equal safety. Tetracaine will produce spinal anaesthesia lasting one and one-half to two hours. Its onset is fairly rapid – five to ten minutes – and the anaesthetic level is invariably "fixed" within twenty minutes. Tetracaine is packaged in ampules containing either 0.2 per cent or 0.3 per cent pontocaine hydrochloride in 6 per cent dextrose solution. These solutions are hyperbaric (s.g. 1.020 to 1.021). Crystals containing 10, 15, 20, and up to 250 mgm are also available. The premixed solutions are recommended.

The level of anaesthesia obtained with tetracaine will vary with the physique of the patient, the site of injection, the rate of injection, the volume of injection, and the positioning of the patient. As a general rule, and using the L 3–4 site of injection, the following anaesthetic levels should be obtained using the tetracaine dosage listed below:

Saddle or perineal block	8–10 mg
T 12	8–10 mg
T 10	10–14 mg
T 8	14–16 mg
T 4	16–20 mg

One should always remember that it is wiser to have the anaesthetic level a little higher than required, rather than a little too low. The tetracaine–glucose spinal technique is the most commonly used, and the most dependable of the agents and techniques available today.

Advantages of Spinal Anaesthesia
Spinal anaesthesia will produce optimum conditions for surgery, i.e., analgesia and muscle relaxation, with the least interference with body function. It is not a difficult technique to master, and can be most valuable to the practising physician providing proper precautions are taken, and patients are carefully and intelligently selected.

Contraindications
The use of spinal anaesthesia is contraindicated in patients with pre-existing neurological disorders, severe shock, severe cardiovascular disease, chronic backache, and preoperative backache. High spinal anaesthesia interferes with the function of the respiratory muscles (abdominal and intercostal) and is contraindicated in patients with respiratory insufficiency.

Care of Patients
Preoperative As a rule, premedication should be heavier than that for general anaesthesia. A barbiturate preparation one and one-half hours preoperatively is also desirable.

Operative (*a*) To prevent undesirable falls in blood pressure, subcutaneous injection of ephedrine (50 mg) may be given half an hour before operation, or at the time of the actual procedure. (*b*) An intravenous infusion should always be in place, in order that supportive therapy by drugs or fluid is easily available. (*c*) Many patients require or request a state of unconsciousness; this is easily produced by an intravenous barbiturate. (*d*) Careful monitoring of the respiration and blood pressure is essential. Oxygen by mask should be readily available, as should vasoconstrictors in case of a fall in blood pressure.

Postoperative The most common postoperative complication is headache, caused by a dural leakage from the spinal tap. As an aid in preventing headache, the use of a small-gauge spinal needle (preferably a no. 26) is recommended, and the patient should be kept supine for 24 hours. The possibility of thermal and pressure injury while the anaesthetic is effective should always be remembered.

EPIDURAL OR PERIDURAL BLOCK

Epidural block is achieved by injecting local anaesthetic solution into the epidural space in the cervical, thoracic, or lumbar area of the vertebral canal. The part-time occasional anaesthetist should limit himself to the lumbar site of injection.

The epidural space lies between the dura mater and the ligaments and periosteum lining the vertebral canal. It extends from the foramen magnum, where the dura fuses with the periosteum of the skull, to the sacrococcygeal membrane. The space is filled with loose areolar tissue, blood vessels, lymphatics, and nerve roots. Local anaesthetic solutions readily pass upwards and downwards through this space.

Solutions Lidocaine (Xylocaine) 1 to 2 per cent, propitocaine (Citanest) 1 to 3 per cent, mepivacaine (Carbocaine) 1 to 2 per cent, and bupivicaine (Marcaine) 0.25 or 0.5 per cent are the local anaesthetic solutions recommended. The total volume used by the occasional anaesthetist should not exceed 15 to 20 cc.

Advantages Epidural block produces anaesthetic conditions somewhat similar to spinal anaesthesia, but without the hazard of headache which may follow the latter technique. It is particularly of value in operations about the vagina and rectum, and especially recommended for obstetrical anaesthesia.

Disadvantages Four disadvantages are: (*a*) difficulty in mastering the technique; (*b*) incomplete anaesthesia: although sensory analgesia may be obtained, motor anaesthesia may not be complete; (*c*) accidental subdural injection of a large volume of local anaesthetic solution, producing a high spinal anaesthetic; (*d*) reaction to the local anaesthetic solution through over-dosage or too rapid absorption.

G.M. WYANT

7
Care of the unconscious patient

Many pathological conditions can cause unconsciousness or coma. While it is true that each different aetiological factor will require specific measures of treatment, the general care of the comatose patient is common to all, whether the state of unconsciousness be due to diabetes, uraemia, a cerebral vascular accident, poisoning, profound cerebral hypoxia, or indeed to anaesthesia. The only difference between anaesthesia and the pathological conditions enumerated is that the unconsciousness of uncomplicated anaesthesia is reversible, whereas this is not assured in pathological states.

At this point it may be useful to consider essential differences between coma and sleep. During sleep the body is still able to take care of its vital interests as it does in the awake state, and thus the viability of the whole is assured. In coma, on the other hand, many vital reflexes are obtunded or entirely in abeyance, and irreparable harm may befall the organism unless the attendant's watchfulness is substituted for some otherwise automatic adjustments. Two simple examples may serve to illustrate this. If during sleep any interference with the blood supply of an extremity occurs and the limb 'goes to sleep,' the individual will awaken and take the necessary action to restore adequate circulation. The comatose patient cannot take such defensive measures, and obstruction of the blood supply will continue to the point of gangrene unless rectified by the intervention of other persons. Or, if 'snoring,' a manifestation of partial obstruction of the airway, causes sufficient cerebral hypoxia, the individual, without necessarily awakening, will change position, thus clearing the airway. Again, no such protective action will be taken by the comatose patient, whose obstruction will continue even if the ensuing asphyxia eventually proves fatal.

It is obvious, then, that in caring for the unconscious individual the physician must make absolutely certain that no harm comes to him and that all functions which were previously controlled by reflex are watched carefully, and all derangements rectified as soon as they occur.

Care of the unconscious patient is best considered under the following headings:

1 Respiratory System;
2 Circulatory System;
3 Physical Factors.

Maintenance of fluid and electrolyte balance and renal function are also of major importance, but can usefully be considered in conjunction with the above systems.

RESPIRATORY SYSTEM

Many of the respiratory factors applicable to the care of the unconscious patient will also be considered in chapter 8 on 'Respiration and Anaesthesia.' Therefore the subjects of apnoea and artificial ventilation will not be covered here, but it must be realized that they are equally applicable to the care of the unconscious.

In the absence of gross pulmonary disease, inadequate ventilation can come about in one of two ways. There may be partial or complete obstruction of the air passages, or the depth of respiration may be inadequate (non-obstructive hypoxia).

Obstructed Respiration
It is axiomatic that noisy respiration is obstructed respiration. Any narrowing of the airway will produce a sound, and that alone is indicative of partial obstruction. This must never be tolerated since

in the long run it will lead to increasing hypoxia and hypercarbia and exhaustion of the muscles of respiration. On the other hand, the corollary does not hold true: absence of sound does not necessarily mean unobstructed respiration. Obviously when the flow of air is interrupted because of complete obstruction, no sound can be produced. Such complete obstruction is characterized by early cyanosis, provided there is an adequate level of haemoglobin, and by 'vertical paradoxical' respiratory movements.

The cause of obstruction may be anatomical (e.g. the base of the tongue) or it may be secretions or blood accumulating anywhere in the respiratory tree, being churned up by the moving column of air. All efforts must be made to re-establish an unobstructed airway. This may be accomplished either by proper positioning of the patient or, if secretions or other foreign materials are at fault, by aspirating them. Mechanical aids such as an oropharyngeal airway or a tracheal tube may be employed where a free airway cannot otherwise be assured. Tracheotomy will relieve any obstruction at the level of the glottis and above and will furthermore permit more thorough and atraumatic repeated aspiration of secretions.

Non-Obstructive Hypoxia
While it is relatively easy to recognize obstruction in any form, and having recognized it, to treat it effectively, the occurrence of underventilation is much more insidious. Cyanosis is not an early sign, and the ensuing hypercarbia will tend to maintain or even to elevate systolic blood pressure and will result in a slow bounding radial pulse. Thus, to the unwary, the patient may give the impression of being in excellent condition. Table I illustrates the problem of underventilation. It is obvious from this that, since the dead space is for all intents and purposes fixed, any reduction in tidal volume will produce a proportionally more significant diminution in alveolar ventilation. If respiratory rate is taken into consideration and a slowing of respiratory rate is postulated in addition to a decreased tidal volume, then the problem will be magnified even further in respect to minute volume. It is obvious that the patient may well be breathing, yet his tidal volume may only clear his dead space and

Table I

Ventilation with reduced respiratory rate

	Normal ventilation	Moderate under-ventilation	Severe under-ventilation
Tidal volume (ml)	500	350	200
Dead space (ml)	150	150	150
Alveolar ventilation (ml)	350	200	50
	RESPIRATORY RATE 20/MIN		
Minute volume (L)	10	7	4
Minute alveolar ventilation (L)	7	4	1
	RESPIRATORY RATE 12/MIN		
Minute volume (L)	6	4.2	2.4
Minute alveolar ventilation (L)	4.2	2.4	0.6

thus alveolar ventilation may be almost entirely absent. This is a lethal situation and the existence of this possibility must be clearly recognized.

While administration of oxygen, with or without artificial ventilation, may be of great importance in all cases where tissue oxygenation is substandard, attention must be paid to adequate humidification of any gases administered. This becomes even more important in the tracheotomized patient where much of the natural humidification mechanism in the nasal and paranasal sinuses is being by-passed. Disregard for this precaution will lead to drying out of the respiratory mucosa, producing thickening of secretions and severe crusting. This, added to suppression of the cough reflex and possibly diminished ciliary activity, may lead to pulmonary atelectasis. Adequate humidification, frequent turning of the patient from side to side, and vigorous physiotherapy will do much to prevent this complication.

If the laryngeal and cough reflexes are obtunded, as is often the case in the unconscious patient, aspiration of stomach contents and of saliva becomes a distinct possibility. There need not necessarily be obvious vomiting; silent regurgitation may occur if the cardiac sphincter is relaxed. Again the lateral position will help to guard against this. If coma is reasonably deep, however, respiratory exchange may be impaired to the point where assistance is required, and in this case a tracheal tube or a tracheotomy will afford the additional advantage of safeguarding against such aspiration.

CIRCULATORY SYSTEM *

In the care of the unconscious patient it is important to realize that cardiovascular homeostasis, like all other reflex activity, is impaired, that adjustments cannot be made efficiently for changes in position, and that vascular tone may be deficient. Treatment aimed at maintenance of circulatory homeostasis is largely symptomatic and devoted to maintenance of adequate tissue perfusion. In order to achieve this, fluid and electrolyte balance must be carefully maintained and adjusted, if they are deranged, and blood or plasma volume expanders may be required. The need for vasopressor agents must be carefully considered from case to case; in the majority of instances not only are they not required but they may even be deleterious to tissue perfusion, although they will maintain or elevate blood pressure as measured in the larger vessels. One of the most reliable indices of adequate tissue perfusion is the urinary output. For this reason every unconscious patient should have an indwelling catheter inserted, and adequate records of intake and output should be maintained. As long as urinary output is adequate, thus indicating adequate renal perfusion, no special measures to maintain blood pressure are indicated. Indeed under some circumstances vasodilator substances may be indicated; although they decrease systemic blood pressure they may improve tissue perfusion. Blood pressure per se is only the rather inaccurate measurement of pressure in the brachial artery at any given time and is not indicative of tissue perfusion, which is the only thing that matters. While the blood pressure cannot be ignored, its significance must never be over-stressed. In any case it must be read in conjunction with other signs of circulatory integrity, such as pulse rate, skin colour, venous filling, and capillary refill-time.

Cardiac output, being in part dependent upon venous return, can be aided by wrapping the legs in elastic bandages and elevating them.

*See also chapter 9, 'Cardiovascular Homeostasis.'

The foot of the bed itself should not be elevated since head-down tilting of the whole body will impair diaphragmatic movement and thus reduce ventilation, and will also impede venous return from the head without substantially increasing total venous return above that obtained by elevating the legs only.

An intravenous infusion with a large-bore needle is set up at an early stage in the management of the patient when veins are still well filled and easily accessible. This will allow unimpeded fluid replacement and intravenous drug administration. In the absence of oral intake, the intravenous route becomes essential for the maintenance of fluid and electrolyte balance and for nutrition. For this reason also, intake and output are continuously charted, and fluids are administered accordingly.

PHYSICAL FACTORS

Since the unconscious patient is unable to protect himself he may suffer physical harm in many ways. He must be so positioned that he will be able to maintain an unobstructed airway and will not be likely to aspirate vomitus. A semi-prone position with the underlying leg flexed to prevent the patient from rolling on his face is the best position. No pillow is allowed.

Great care must be taken to protect all anatomically vulnerable points such as the external peroneal nerve at the fibular head, the radial nerve in the radial groove and the brachial plexus, by proper positioning and padding. Careful skin management is necessary to prevent pressure sores, and hot water bottles must be used with extreme caution since burns may easily be caused through the patient's inability to withdraw from noxious stimuli. Frequent turning from side to side is important to allow more even pulmonary ventilation and to prevent pressure sores. The corneae must be protected from drying and from abrasion, and pressure on the eye must be avoided. The patient must be protected from falling out of bed, and bedside rails must always be in position.

From the foregoing it will easily be appreciated that the care of the unconscious patient is an onerous task which requires constant attention to detail.

When an unconscious patient is first seen, the following steps should be undertaken:

Emergency Procedures

1 Ascertain the adequacy of respiratory exchange and, if necessary, assist respiration or institute artificial respiration.

2 Ascertain the adequacy of circulation by palpation of pulses, testing for capillary refill time, and taking the blood pressure. Take action as indicated, including artificial circulation. An electrocardiogram may be needed at this early stage, but treatment is not to be delayed because it is not immediately available.

3 Institute an intravenous infusion with a large-bore needle for future use.

Diagnosis

4 Attempt to get a history from the patient's relatives or friends.

5 Proceed with a thorough physical examination, with special reference to neurological tests.

6 Insert a self-retaining urethral catheter. Obtain specimens of urine and blood for laboratory analysis to exclude possibilities of diabetes, uraemia, etc. If barbiturate poisoning is suspected, barbiturate blood levels may be determined. Lumbar puncture will exclude subarachnoid haemorrhage and other central nervous system diseases.

7 Take such X-rays as are indicated to confirm diagnosis.

Definitive Procedure

8 If assistance in ventilation is required, manual assistance may now be replaced by a mechanical ventilator.

9 Obtain a baseline of the depth of coma by charting various reflexes and recording the electroencephalogram. This may be repeated from time to time to record progress.

10 Order daily chest films.

11 Institute antibiotic therapy.

12 Take every measure to combat the specific cause of the coma.

13 Institute fluid intake and output charts, and write intake orders based on laboratory findings and clinical requirements.

14 See that frequent changes in position are made.

15 Undertake symptomatic treatment to maintain adequate tissue perfusion. This will include wrapping and elevation of the legs if necessary, and the administration of vasodilator or vasoconstrictor substances.

16 Make sure vulnerable points are protected; the corneas should be moistened repeatedly.

17 Institute skin and mouth care.

18 Record body temperature and treat hyperpyrexia, if it occurs, by standard means.

H.B.F. FAIRLEY

8
Respiration and anaesthesia

The respiratory mechanism is concerned with four related functions: (*a*) delivery of oxygen from ambient atmosphere to cells; (*b*) elimination of carbon dioxide in the reverse direction; (*c*) maintenance of acid-base balance; (*d*) maintenance of venous return. Each of these functions may be deranged in patients coming to the operating room, and may be disturbed during anaesthesia and surgery or in the postoperative period.

PREOPERATIVE ASSESSMENT OF RESPIRATORY STATUS

For purposes of description and assessment, pulmonary function may be divided artificially into components: (*a*) oxygen consumption and CO_2 production per unit time; (*b*) ventilation, involving volume exchange of air and the mechanics of this exchange; (*c*) the quantitative relationships between ventilation of alveoli and their perfusion with pulmonary capillary blood; (*d*) diffusion involving the passage of respiratory gases across the alveolar membrane; (*e*) gas transport mechanisms in blood. Each may be quantitated, and the possible tests are numerous. An outline of the more relevant measurements follows, but these will always complement a careful history and physical examination, in which a history of exertional dyspnoea, of orthopnoea, of asthmatic attacks, of quantity and colour of sputum, and any history suggesting cardiac failure will be of chief interest. Direct questioning will elicit therapeutic history, with particular reference to bronchodilators and their efficacy, steroids, diuretics, digitalis, and antibiotics. Physical findings are difficult to correlate with pulmonary function figures but should assist in the overall determination of whether respiratory disability is sufficient to merit further evaluation. To some extent, this decision will be influenced by the nature of the intended surgery. Thus, upper abdominal and thoracic surgery involves considerably more hazard to such patients than simple procedures on a limb, which may be handled with regional anaesthesia.

Ventilation

Two types of ventilatory defect exist: restrictive and obstructive. The former is peculiar to all persons unable to take a big breath, whether because of inability to perform respiratory muscular work (e.g. post-poliomyelitis) or because of increased elastic opposition to this work (e.g. rigid chest wall, as with kyphoscoliosis; or stiff lung, as with pulmonary fibrosis). Obstructive defects are due to narrowed lower airways, the most common cause being the expiratory air-trapping associated with emphysema.

These defects are obviously of interest to the anaesthetist and are easily measured by the Timed Vital Capacity or Forced Expiratory Volume in One Second (F.E.V.$_1$). Tables (dependent on height and weight) are available for normal values for Vital Capacity. The patient takes a maximum inspiration, followed by a maximum expiration. The latter is the Vital Capacity. When this is done as rapidly as possible, over 75 per cent of this 'forced expiratory volume' should be expired in the first second if there is no obstructive defect.

A further test of ventilation is the Maximum Voluntary Ventilation (M.V.V.), the maximum volume the patient can move in one minute's hyperventilation. This is usually performed over 15 seconds and multiplied by 4. Since patients with restriction can take rapid short breaths, this is mainly a test of airway patency. If F.E.V. or M.V.V. is low, the response to bronchodilator should be assessed.

Should there be a pronounced ventilatory defect, arterial blood should be examined to determine whether there is any carbon dioxide retention. Normal values for arterial carbon dioxide tension (Pa_{CO_2}) are 38 to 42 mm Hg. Should Pa_{CO_2} be elevated, a respiratory acidosis is said to be present and an arterial pH value will indicate whether this is uncompensated (acute) or compensated (chronic).

Arterial Po_2 (Pa_{O_2}) also varies with ventilation but, unlike the Pa_{CO_2}, is dependent upon other factors and is therefore not such a useful ventilatory index.

The vast majority of chronic respiratory disorders in patients coming to the operating room will be exposed by the simple tests mentioned. Occasionally there is no disorder of ventilation, despite arterial oxygen desaturation. This situation is usually due to ventilation/perfusion inequality.

Ventilation-Perfusion Relationships
The determination of ventilation-perfusion relationships involves moderately complex concepts and measurements, many of which are not appropriate to routine evaluation of pulmonary function. However, the concepts are important to the anaesthetist. Essentially, if any particular alveolus is not ventilated and perfused in the usual relationship of 4 to 5, one of two disorders may arise: (*a*) unperfused alveoli, the volume of which constitutes alveolar dead-space. Unless total minute volume is increased proportionately, alveolar ventilation will fall and CO_2 retention will result. (*b*) Diminished ventilation, relative to perfusion, results in mixed venous blood being transferred to the arterial circulation in an inadequately oxygenated form.

Note that this venous admixture effect cannot be corrected by hyperventilation, owing to the non-linear uptake of oxygen by blood. Once fully saturated, blood perfusing the adequately ventilated alveoli will accept very little additional oxygen during hyperventilation. This is in distinction to the relatively linear carbon dioxide dissociation curve, which permits compensation for 'shunted' carbon dioxide by hyperventilation of other alveoli. It should also be noted that, although hyperventilation in the sense of an increased minute ventilation will not correct venous admixture effect, large tidal ventilation may be effective in expanding atelectatic areas and this manoeuvre is a useful adjunct to other forms of chest physical therapy.

Usually some degree of both venous admixture and dead-space effects is present, and since most patients can hyperventilate in compensation, the common residual finding will be an abnormally low arterial oxygen tension. (Note also that the venous admixture effect will produce a low diffusing capacity figure and accounts for many apparent abnormalities of diffusion.)

Diffusion

Since CO_2 diffuses twenty times as rapidly as oxygen, diffusion is for all intents and purposes a problem of oxygen transfer. Diffusion defects are nearly always associated with other disorders of pulmonary function but may, rarely, occur on their own. Total oxygen diffusion is dependent upon a number of variables responsible for maintaining an oxygen tension gradient between the alveoli and the pulmonary capillary blood. These include the inspired oxygen tension, ventilation, and cardiac output, among others. The diffusing capacity for any particular gas is the quantity of that gas diffusing from alveoli to blood per minute per mm Hg gradient and thus, theoretically, the expression ignores factors other than those in the alveolar-capillary membrane. In practice, it is probable that diffusing capacity measurements serve to measure two other major factors, ventilation/perfusion inequality and pulmonary capillary blood volume. It is therefore decreased after pulmonary resection, in emphysema and in a variety of disorders producing so-called alveolar-capillary block (but probably due to associated ventilation/perfusion inequality), e.g. sarcoidosis, berylliosis, carcinomatosis, pulmonary fibrosis.

Gas Transport

Two major distinctions exist between the respiratory roles of oxygen and carbon dioxide, having quite different clinical implications.

1 *Carriage* Since oxygen is carried predominantly in combination with haemoglobin, the shape of the oxyhaemoglobin dissociation

curve is most important. The major practical implication is that, as arterial oxygen tension falls, saturation (and therefore content) falls minimally until the shoulder of the curve is reached at tensions of approximately 50 mm Hg (Fig. 1). The slope of the curve then

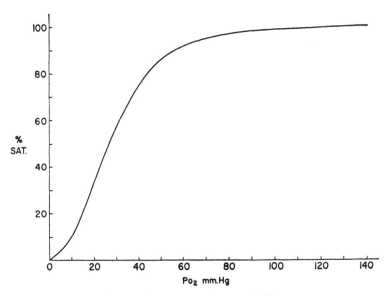

FIGURE 1 Oxygen dissociation curve for haemoglobin

changes from relatively horizontal to relatively vertical, so that a further fall in tension produces a rapid desaturation. This accounts for the apparent reserve seen clinically followed by 'sudden' distress. The carbon dioxide dissociation curve is more linear and the same 'shoulder' does not exist.

2. *Gas stores* The vast majority of the body's oxygen store is in the blood, in combination with haemoglobin. Very little oxygen is present in the tissues at any one time. The total store in the average adult is of the order of 1000 ml, which is consumed at the rate of 200 to 300 ml/min. The immediate consequences of apnoea or of oxygen withdrawal are obvious. Carbon dioxide stores are vast,

being present in all tissues and amounting to several litres, of which much is available to the HCO_3 buffer system. In the event of ventilatory depression or of 'apnoeic oxygenation,' CO_2 is slowly stored and Pa_{CO_2} rises at the rate of 3–4 mm Hg each minute.

VENTILATION DURING ANAESTHESIA

Metabolism and, therefore, oxygen consumption and carbon dioxide production are reduced during general anaesthesia. However, in addition, the central control of ventilation is depressed by narcotics, barbiturates, and most inhalation anaesthetic agents, the most notable exception being nitrous oxide. In consequence the average premedicated patient, breathing spontaneously under general anaesthesia, under-ventilates relative to the demands of tissue metabolism, in proportion to depth of anaesthesia. Under-ventilation occurs at lighter levels with certain agents, particularly halothane, forane, and cyclopropane. When abdominal relaxation is achieved by deep anaesthesia or by the use of muscle relaxants, the degree of under-ventilation will be such as to make mechanical assistance necessary.

In addition to the patient's general disinclination to breathe under anaesthesia, the respiratory work requirements are frequently increased as a result of increases in dead-space and in airway resistance. Increases in dead-space may be mechanical (e.g., masks or circuits with inadequate flow elimination of expired gases) or alveolar (i.e., inspired air moving in and out of unperfused alveoli; this is a common occurrence during anaesthesia and has been shown to be inversely proportional to the depression in cardiac output – and, probably, in pulmonary artery pressure – occurring with most general anaesthetics). These problems may be minimized by careful attention to circuits and flows and by tracheal intubation. Increases in resistance may be minimized by using as wide tubing as possible in circuits, by using wide-bore tracheal tubes and connectors, and by avoiding valves with high resistances.

Ventilation may be assessed during anaesthesia by measurement of tidal volume with a simple meter (such as the Wright Anemometer). Values obtained can be compared with normal figures from the Radford nomogram, which indicates normal values for tidal volume at various combinations of body weight and respiratory rate.

For the reasons outlined above, it will be necessary on many occasions to use mechanical ventilation. This usually takes the form of positive pressure intermittently applied to the upper airway. The amount of pressure required is mainly a function of the elastic recoil of the lungs and chest wall and of the resistance to air flow offered by the upper and lower airways. Ideally, one should adjust the pressure to deliver an adequate measured tidal volume. In patients with a near normal blood volume and functionally intact cardio-vascular system, intermittent positive pressure ventilation will not produce sufficient change in intrathoracic pressure to cause a physiologically important drop in venous return, cardiac output, or systemic blood pressure – provided the expiratory phase of the respiratory cycle is at least as long as inspiration and preferably longer. The occasional emphysematous patient with marked air trapping furnishes an exception to this rule.

CHOICE OF ANAESTHETIC IN PATIENTS WITH RESPIRATORY DISEASE

All patients for elective surgery should come to the operating room in optimum condition, following physiotherapy and antibiotics for sputum reduction, bronchodilators, steroids, or cardiotonics should these be indicated. It is possible to document the fact that, in the absence of such preoperative preparation, mean length of hospital stay is increased because of postoperative complications and, rarely, mortality is increased.

Regional or General Anaesthesia
The decision to use a regional or general anaesthetic will depend on operative site when balanced against the severity of the pulmonary function problem. Upper abdominal or thoracic procedures in patients with severe ventilatory defects should be handled with a technique permitting ventilatory assistance. The underlying prin-

ciple will be the avoidance of potent respiratory depressants, of bronchoconstrictors, and of agents not permitting early arousal. Halothane has been shown to produce bronchodilatation, as have diethyl ether and methoxyflurane. However, early arousal is most easily achieved after halothane.

Spontaneous or Controlled Ventilation

The respiratory depression inherent in general anaesthesia with spontaneous respiration is particularly to be avoided in patients with serious ventilatory defects, particularly of the obstructive type. Many of those with chronic CO_2 retention are somewhat dependent upon mild hypoxaemia for their respiratory drive, and this may be a further cause of under-ventilation when they are presented with the high oxygen tensions common (and desirable) in inhalation anaesthesia.

Controlled respiration, using muscle relaxants and very light anaesthesia, permits early awakening and usually ensures adequate volume exchange. The problem most frequently encountered is in the very small group of patients with severe air trapping, in whom volume exchange may be difficult and in whom the raised intrathoracic pressures may impede venous return and produce a fall in blood pressure. In such patients, trial and error using different inspired pressures and inspiratory-expiratory durations – along with measurement of ventilatory volumes and venous systemic blood pressure – may be the only recourse.

VENOUS ADMIXTURE DURING ANAESTHESIA

A reduction in resting lung volume is common during anaesthesia, particularly in spontaneously breathing obese patients. This is associated with an increase in venous admixture. In addition, a reduction in cardiac output (over and above that due to reduction in metabolic rate) is common. The resulting mixed venous desaturation (for any given degree of intrapulmonary shunting) causes further arterial desaturation. Consequently, it is customary to give at least 35 per cent inspired oxygen during anaesthesia and, in any case of doubt, to measure arterial oxygen tension.

Controlled ventilation with large tidal volumes is a useful prophylactic manoeuvre in the maintenance of resting lung volume.

POSTOPERATIVE RESPIRATORY PROBLEMS

A separate chapter is devoted to this issue. However, certain of the problems described as occurring during anaesthesia may persist or even be accentuated in the recovery phase.

1 *Hypoxia* A low arterial oxygen tension is extremely common in the postoperative period. Since cyanosis is not usually evident until tensions have fallen to half normal values, this may be extremely difficult to detect clinically, although it may contribute to hypotension and restlessness, for example.

Consequently, oxygen administration should be routine in the immediate postoperative period. In the rare patient with respiratory disease severe enough to produce CO_2 retention, ventilatory volumes and, if necessary, blood gases should be monitored, lest high oxygen tensions produce respiratory depression.

The causes of this hypoxaemia may be various. Most importantly, the miliary atelectasis described as occurring in many patients during anaesthesia persists at least until the patient rouses, becomes at least partially mobile in bed, and begins to take large breaths. Similarly, the mixed venous desaturation (reflected on the arterial side through any shunt), caused by depressed cardiac output, persists for a variable period depending upon the elimination of the causative agents.

Recovery of the various organ systems from the effects of anaesthesia and surgery does not necessarily occur at the same rate. Thus, muscle tone and shivering may be quite vigorous at a time when ventilation and cardiac output cannot keep pace. The net result will be hypoxaemia and anaerobic glycolysis.

After the more major surgical operations, persisting hypovolaemia may also cause a reduction in cardiac output, with resulting mixed venous desaturation and its possible arterial consequences.

2 *Under-ventilation* Satisfactory ventilation depends on the proper balance of a triad of circumstances:

Metabolic ventilatory demand

$\downarrow$ $\uparrow$

Intact central mechanism $\longrightarrow$ Ability to perform muscular work against thoraco-pulmonary resistance and dead-space

Occasionally an imbalance arises because of situations such as metabolic acidosis, central depression, persistence of curarization, pulmonary pathology, or various combinations – with resulting under-ventilation.

Following the use of controlled ventilation during the operative period, the return to spontaneous ventilation is usually uneventful. However, it is always necessary to assess the adequacy of the spontaneous volumes and, if any doubt exists, to measure tidal volume and frequency, arterial blood gas tensions and pH. If the patient is co-operative, the vital capacity will indicate the degree of his ventilatory reserve. Thirty to fifty per cent of predicted normal is very acceptable at this time and volumes less than 10 ml/kg strongly suggest continued ventilation until the situation is evaluated further. The further evaluation may include degree of persisting myoneural block; pulmonary status clinically and radiologically; cardiovascular status, clinically, electrocardiographically, and haemodynamically; level of persisting central nervous system depression; blood volume, clinically including balance records and haematocrit and, if necessary, by weighing and indicator dilution studies; acid-base and electrolyte balance. If in doubt, the guiding principle is to maintain ventilation and oxygenation until it is obvious that all relevant organ systems are stable and there is some indication (particularly from vital capacity and inspired-arterial oxygen tension difference) that spontaneous respiration is likely to be satisfactorily maintained. In the more complex situations, a trial period of spontaneous respiration through the tracheal tube may then be advisable.

It has now become common practice, if not routine, to ventilate certain patients 'prophylactically' for several hours postoperatively. Examples include many patients who have undergone cardiac surgery, who may have a low cardiac output, an unstable cardiac rhythm, persistent bleeding, and/or left atrial hypertension and pulmonary oedema. Emergency surgery for major trauma or major abdominal or thoracic catastrophes may be handled similarly. The common feature is a situation which is sufficiently unstable physiologically to require fully efficient ventilation and oxygenation, in order to avoid compounding the problem.

PAUL E. OTTON

9

Cardiovascular homeostasis in relation to anaesthesia and resuscitation

The cardiovascular system is well endowed to adapt to the varying demands of the body, and so keep the conditions in the internal environment constant. This constant balance of conditions is known as homeostasis. Anaesthesia unavoidably moderates this response, narrowing the range of adaptation. The study of the effects of anaesthetics is as much concerned with this influence on homeostasis as it is with the anaesthetic state. It is the aim of this chapter to outline the way in which anaesthesia affects cardiovascular homeostasis, and to indicate when resuscitation is necessary to assist nature in regaining control.

PHYSIOLOGICAL CONSIDERATIONS

At its simplest, the circulation consists of a low-pressure, high-capacity venous reservoir feeding blood to a central pump, and a high-pressure, low-capacity arterial system that partitions the total output of the pump according to the local needs of the tissues. The cardiovenous unit safeguards the survival of the organism as a whole, whereas the arterial system protects individual organs.

The total body blood flow or cardiac output is dependent on the functional integrity of two components of the cardiovascular system; the contractile venous reservoir and the pump.

Venous return, or the rate of blood flow into the heart is determined by a balance between the capacity of the venous reservoir, as set by the peripheral venous tone, and the circulating blood volume. Venous tone varies the circulatory capacity, shrinking or expanding the container to fit the volume of any given moment, and so maintains a constant driving pressure for returning blood to the heart.

The pumping action of the heart translates venous return into cardiac output. The balance between the volume of venous return and the ability of the right heart to pump blood establishes the right auricular pressure. This pressure is more easily measured as the central venous pressure (C.V.P.) and serves as a convenient monitor of the efficiency with which the pump can handle the returned blood.

The ability of a patient to survive surgical stress, trauma and anaesthesia is greatly dependent on the capacity of the cardio-circulation to sustain a sufficient flow of oxygenated blood to meet the demands of every tissue. If an adequate cardiac output cannot be maintained, either through failure of venous return or an ineffective pump, then circulatory failure exists. Chronically, this defect is termed heart failure, and acutely it is circulatory shock.

The function of cardiac output is to perfuse the tissues. Alteration in arteriole tone, by changing the resistance in response to local tissue needs, regulates the distribution of tissue perfusion and determines the perfusing pressure.

The homeostatic integration of these cardiovascular responses depends on an intact autonomic nervous system, particularly the sympatho-adrenal system, and reactive cardiac and vascular muscle.

The basic cardiovascular effect of all anaesthesia is to depress the contractile components directly as well as to alter the body's ability for reflex neurohumeral compensation. The interference with reflex compensation appears to originate within the central nervous system and is affected by anaesthetics in different ways. One type, represented by halothane and methoxyflurane, would appear to depress all levels of central reflex control. The other, represented by cyclopropane, selectively releases the vasomotor facilitatory neurones with an over-all increase in sympathetic activity. Both general and conduction anaesthesia damp the normal mechanisms for cardiovascular homeostasis.

A reduced cardiac output is the significant alteration involved, and is due to two main changes. Primarily there is a decrease in venous return, as a result of expansion of the vascular bed due to reduced venomotor tone. Secondly, depression of myocardial function impairs the ability of the heart to convert venous return into cardiac output. In addition, most halogenated anaesthetics and cyclopropane sensitize the myocardium to adrenaline-induced arrhythmias, the extreme form of which is ventricular fibrillation.

The effect of an individual anaesthetic agent depends upon the rate, depth, and duration of administration, and the ability of the circulation to respond. Pre-existing diseases associated with a high peripheral vascular tone, either as a cause or as a compensation, are most prone to anaesthetic influence.

Patients with *arterial hypertension* will have profound falls in blood pressure whenever peripheral resistance is reduced by anaesthesia. Potent anti-hypertensive medical therapy may interact to increase the anaesthetic embarrassment.

Cardiac insufficiency with a low and relatively fixed cardiac output from valvular, myocardial, or pericardial disease depends on an intact responsive peripheral circulation for compensation. It is common for anaesthesia to disturb this compensation.

Hypovolaemia from haemorrhage and fluid loss can temporarily be compensated by contraction of the peripheral vascular container. Anaesthesia can readily undo this compensation.

The safety of any individual anaesthetic agent depends greatly on the skill with which it is administered and the accuracy with which it is tailored to the response of the patient. There are, nevertheless, sufficiently consistent differences between the various agents to warrant their separate consideration.

REGIONAL, SPINAL, AND EPIDURAL ANALGESIA

The main cardiovascular effects of regional, spinal, and epidural analgesia follow on the coincident unavoidable sympathetic paralysis, the extent of which determines the degree of haemodynamic disturbance. Sympathetic blockade below the fourth thoracic nerve root denervates peripheral vascular smooth muscle. Denervation of the arterioles reduces peripheral resistance and promotes hypotension. Denervation of the veins increases their capacity, creating an unfavourable balance with circulating blood volume, diminishing venous return and hence cardiac output. Head-down posturing and adequate fluid volume replacement will promote the recovery of venous return.

Extension of regional block above the fifth thoracic root adds the further handicap of sympathetic denervation of the heart. Myocardial contractile response is reduced, while the intact vagal tone promotes bradycardia. The haemodynamic consequence of a severe reduction in cardiac output coupled with an unresponsive arteriolar resistance system is profound hypotension.

Vasomotor drugs that reduce venous capacity, increase arterial resistance, and directly stimulate the myocardium will effectively replace the loss from sympathetic paralysis. Noradrenaline (Levophed®), mephentermine (Wyamine®), methamphetamine (Methedrine®), and metarmine (Aramine®) are among the most effective.

GENERAL ANAESTHETICS

Intravenous Agents
Much of the recent progress in general anaesthesia has come about through the development of intravenous drugs with more specific pharmacological activity.

Barbiturates – thiopentone, methohexitone, etc. The fatal ease with which an overdose of intravenous barbiturate can be given to a patient constitutes their greatest hazard. When used prudently to induce light anaesthesia these drugs are as well and as safely tolerated as other agents. The major effect on haemodynamics is to reduce venomotor tone, expand the vascular bed and reduce venous return. Direct myocardial depression will also occur with greater dosage. Patients whose haemodynamics are compensated by a high peripheral vascular tone are most susceptible to these effects of barbiturates.

Narcotic analgesics In clinical dosage the cardiovascular effects of narcotic analgesics are not unlike those produced by some of the barbiturates. The relatively lower doses used solely for supplemental analgesia usually limit any profound circulatory changes. Morphine appears to be especially well tolerated by the resting cardiovascular system, possibly because of coincidental adrenergic stimulation. Recently it has been reintroduced in supraclinical doses and, when combined with proper ventilation and oxygen, is a safe, sole maintenance agent.

Neuroleptanaesthesia This peculiar state of anaesthesia is produced by the combined effect of a narcotic analgesic and a major tranquillizer. The original combination of meperidine and chlorpromazine was an attempt to produce artificial hibernation. Recently more specific agents have been developed, the most popular of which is phenoperidine (Droperidol®), and a short-acting narcotic, fentanyl, combined in a fixed ratio as Innovar®.

Cardiovascular depressant effects exist but are minimized by a slow (half-hour) induction. The major circulatory effects are vasodilatation (adrenergic blockade) and tachycardia with a stable cardiac rhythm. There is potentiation of the circulatory effects of any co-existing hypovolaemia; therefore its use should be combined with liberal volume replacement.

Ketamine This agent provides an interesting departure from orthodox general anaesthesia. The anaesthetic state produced is a type of akinetic cataplexy, but with analgesia. Consciousness is only superficially lost while airway control and ventilation are maintained. The cardiovascular effects are stimulatory, possibly through central vasomotor excitation, producing significant increases in blood pressure with tachycardia.

Diazepam (Valium) This drug is not a primary anaesthetic agent but it is widely used for its sedative and hypnotic properties either given alone to produce amnesia or in combination with regional analgesia. A unique cardiovascular effect is a stabilizing influence on cardiac arrhythmias making it particularly useful in electrical cardioversion procedures.

Inhalation Anaesthetics

Nitrous oxide The simplest and most inert of all anaesthetic agents and, providing oxygenation is adequate, exerts little direct effect on the cardiovascular system. This feature is of value in states of low cardiovascular tolerance. However, its lack of potency requires that it be supplemented for greater depth of anaesthetic control and the supplements are capable of exerting more profound cardiovascular effects.

Diethyl ether Characterized by having its direct cardiovascular depression offset, in part, by a strong sympathetic stimulation. Cardiac efficiency is reduced, but cardiac output and blood pressure are well maintained in light anaesthesia. Tachycardia, with a stable rhythm, is consistent. The apparent safety of ether is dependent on its slowness to effect changes and the support of these changes by increased sympathetic activity. Both of these features may become disadvantageous after prolonged use and during recovery.

Cyclopropane A potent and rapid direct toxin to the cardiovascular system. However, an intact sympatho-adrenal system is strongly stimulated to preserve or accentuate vascular contraction. This increase in peripheral arteriole tone supports arterial blood pressure at normal levels or higher, even in the face of a reduced cardiac output. In clinical conditions of hypovolaemia this property can be of value as a temporary crutch for the blood pressure, if it is borne in mind that cyclopropane acts in this way at the expense of visceral perfusion. The heart rate is typically slow, but the myocardium is more irritable and sensitive to adrenaline. Hence cardiac arrhythmias are common. Carbon dioxide excess accentuates the cardiovascular effects and respiratory depression is unavoidable with cyclopropane anaesthesia under spontaneous respiration. During recovery from cyclopropane the anaesthetic depression often outlasts the sympathetic prop and hypotension occurs frequently enough to be termed 'cyclopropane shock.'

Halothane (Fluothane) A potent, rapid-acting anaesthetic that features a broad flattening of homeostatic reflexes. It produces the direct vascular muscle depression common with other agents. This depression is further promoted by the lowering of central sympathetic vasomotor support which allows the direct cardiovascular effects to obtain significance. Parasympathetic activity is retained and becomes dominant, leading to bradycardia. Cardiac efficiency and output are reduced and this reduction, linked with a low peripheral resistance, leads to some degree of hypotension. Ventricular irritability is heightened and the heart is sensitized to adrenaline.

Chloroform Remarkably similar to halothane, but more potent in cause and effect. Historically it has an unfavourable reputation for serious cardiac and hepatic effects which restrict its present-day use.

Trichlorethylene (Trilene) Has potent toxic cardiac effects if used for total anaesthesia. When restricted to low concentrations for analgesia alone, or to supplement other agents, it exerts minimal effects. Myocardial sensitization to adrenaline and carbon dioxide is present at all concentrations.

Methoxyflurane (Penthrane) Even more effective than halothane in blocking the sympathetic response required to compensate for the direct vascular depression. Cardiac output is reduced, and blood pressure will not be supported by an increase in peripheral resistance especially in deeper planes of anaesthesia.

MUSCLE RELAXANTS

The advent of specific muscle relaxants has resulted in significant reduction in the depth of anaesthesia required for many surgical procedures and coincident with it there has been a sparing of cardiovascular depression. Present-day relaxants exert no specific, direct cardiovascular effects. Secondary effects on the circulation come about either through partial blocking of autonomic ganglion transmission or electrolyte shifts across the muscle membrane.

Gallamine (Flaxedil) Specifically blocks the cardiac vagus to produce tachycardia.

Succinylcholine Usually exerts little influence on the cardiocirculation. However, under exceptional pathophysiological circumstances the effects may be catastrophic. Severe catabolic states, as may subacutely follow extensive surface burns, muscle trauma and denervation (paraplegia), can respond to succinylcholine by the excessive release of intracellular potassium into the circulation in quantities sufficient to produce cardiac arrest. Furthermore, repeat doses within short intervals in normal individuals, particularly infants, may cause profound bradycardia to the point of asystole. These profound cardiovascular actions contraindicate the use of succinylcholine under these exceptional circumstances.

D-tubocurarine Is in itself devoid of direct action on the cardiovascular system. Potent but transient secondary effects from autonomic ganglion blockade may follow large intravenous doses. The haemodynamic consequences of this blockade are most pronounced when large doses of curare are combined with general anaesthetics that also dampen sympathetic compensation (halothane, methoxyflurane) or when hypovolaemia co-exists.

Pancuronium (Pavulon) A recently introduced competitive muscle relaxant virtually devoid of significant autonomic effects, it will obviate many of the present circulatory disadvantages of curare.

However, the major effects of all muscle relaxants on the cardiovascular system follow the use of positive pressure respiration, a mandatory technique whenever muscle relaxants are given. The reversal of intrathoracic pressure from negative to positive displaces blood into the peripheral veins. An intact responsive venous system will limit the volume displaced and maintain venous return. Deep anaesthesia or extensive sympathetic paralysis destroys the normal compensation for these impedances and allows blood to be pooled in the periphery away from the heart. The tolerance of this volume shift is much less when hypovolaemia is present.

Hypothermia
Moderate total body cooling to 30° C decreases the force of myocardial contractions and the heart rate. The heart is more irritable and ventricular fibrillation may occur but is most likely below 29° C. Cardiac output and blood pressure are reduced, but the tissue per-

fusion is sufficient to maintain the reduced demands of tissue metabolism.

Induced Hypotension

Ganglionic and adrenergic blocking agents reduce sympathetic vasomotor control over the peripheral vessels, but have no effect on the
myocardium. Hypotension and a reduction in tissue blood flow
make for a relatively bloodless operating field, a valuable condition
in certain types of surgery.

MONITORING OF THE CARDIOVASCULAR SYSTEM

The proper conduct of any anaesthetic demands simple but constant
contact with the patient's cardiovascular system. The extent of this
contact depends on the pre-existing condition of the patient and the
anticipated anaesthetic or surgical procedure. The time-honoured
observations of pulse, blood pressure, and skin perfusion suffice in
most instances. From these measurements fairly accurate predictions
of a more sophisticated nature can be made.

Direct arterial palpation Can be conveniently complemented by a
stethoscope strapped to the precordium. This method provides a
simple and constant monitor of heart rate and rhythm.

Arterial blood pressure Is usually recorded by the classic methods
of palpation or auscultation. The most accurate and satisfactory
display of the arterial pressure is provided by direct arterial can-
nulation and is most valuable in states of low perfusion and a narrow
pulse pressure.

The central venous pressure Is an invaluable index when more detailed cardiovascular contact is required. It is measured by means
of a small venous catheter advanced into the chest, or by a needle
in the external jugular vein, pressure being recorded by a simple
saline manometer. The central venous pressure is a measure of the
ability of the right heart to handle the blood it receives from the
periphery. The latter, in turn, is a result of the balance between
blood volume and the tone of venous reservoir. The central venous

pressure thus integrates three important parameters: myocardial function, blood volume, and vascular capacity.

A low central venous pressure with arterial hypotension points to a disparity between the vascular system and its filling volume. Refilling of the vascular bed with whole blood or volume expanders will raise the arterial pressure and slow the pulse, while the central venous pressure remains within the normal limits of 5–15 cm saline. This response is a more valid index of adequate volume replacement than is a knowledge of the actual blood volume. If the vascular system is known to be dilated as a result of anaesthetic sympathetic blockade, balance can best be achieved by shrinking the system to normal with vasopressors to better fit the blood volume.

A high or rising venous pressure following volume replacement, without a good response of the pulse and arterial pressure, indicates a failure of the heart to pump the blood that is returned to it. Attention is then focused on the correction of the cardiac inefficiency.

The electrocardiogram Preferably using the oscilloscope, serves as a continuous monitor of the electrical activity of the heart. It is of greatest value in the diagnosis of cardiac arrhythmias and assists in the diagnosis of ischaemia, but it is of no use in measuring the performance of the heart as a pump. Unfortunately, it is possible to depress the heart to the point of asystole without altering the gross appearance of the electrocardiogram.

Blood volume Accurate estimates of blood volume can now be made quickly, but as with other single measurements, these must be integrated with the rest of the circulatory parameters. A determination of blood volume tells only how much is in the container, and nothing of how much the container should hold for any given situation, or how well the pump can handle this volume.

Cardiac output The single most important parameter of the circulatory system, it best reflects the integration of cardiovascular dynamics. Adequate rapid bedside determinations of this most valuable information are still not available. In the past, this lack has led to an over-reliance on arterial blood pressure as the index of an adequate circulation. Therefore treatment has tended to stress control of blood pressure rather than tissue perfusion. The more frequent use of cardiac output determinations will serve to direct attention to blood flow as the measure of cardiovascular function.

Biochemical monitoring The success with which the circulation maintains an adequate tissue perfusion is reflected in the degree of tissue hypoxia that develops. A low blood pH and a depressed buffer base with an accumulation of lactic acid is a measure of the extent of hypoxia due to failure of perfusion.

The circulatory effects of a low pH are depression of the myocardium and dilatation of peripheral vessels, resulting in further reduction of cardiac output and arterial pressure. Failure of respiratory compensation occurs under anaesthesia, leading to a high carbon dioxide tension or hypoxia, both of which will increase the circulatory depression. The low pH can be controlled by assuring adequate respiratory compensation and replacement of buffer base by bicarbonate.

CARDIOVASCULAR HOMEOSTASIS IN RESUSCITATION

Cardiovascular resuscitation is necessary whenever the cardiac output falls below levels sufficient to maintain adequate tissue vitality. Acute failure of cardiac output is termed circulatory shock and in surgical patients is most frequently due to hypovolaemia from blood loss. The need for resuscitation parallels the degree of output depression and reaches its ultimate in cardiac standstill. For the anaesthetist cardiovascular resuscitation revolves around the management of hypovolaemic shock and cardiac standstill.

Cardiac Standstill

Cardiac standstill is the cessation of an adequate heart beat and is of two distinct types: asystole and ventricular fibrillation. The type and extent of any underlying heart disease; the nature of the surgical procedures, especially if it includes a direct attack on the heart or involves a large loss of blood and the type and skill of anaesthetic management are the factors that interplay in the aetiology of cardiac arrest in the operating theatre.

Both fibrillation and asystole result in the absence of a cardiac output, the main immediate danger of which is irreversible cerebral damage. This insult begins within three minutes of circulatory arrest and by eight minutes produces damage that is incompatible with long-term survival. The immediate diagnosis and resuscitation of the circulation is thus vital.

The only reliable diagnostic signs of the lack of cardiac output are the absence of pulse, blood pressure, and peripheral blood flow. The electrocardiogram may delay diagnosis of asystole by showing persistent electrical activity of the heart.

Once the diagnosis is confirmed the treatment is by two simultaneous steps; (*a*) artificial ventilation of the lungs, preferably with 100 per cent oxygen; (*b*) restoration of an effective circulation by cardiac compression.

If a direct current electrical defibrillator is immediately available, even if the diagnosis is not clear, it is worthwhile applying a single external shock initially in the hope that an early ventricular fibrillation may be quickly converted. If ineffective, immediate rhythmic cardiac compression must be commenced.

Artificial circulation by cardiac compression (cardiac massage) is established by one of two methods:

1 *Closed chest technique* This is the simplest, most rapid method of restoring an effective cardiac output. It is done with the patient in the supine position on a firm surface such as the operating table, the floor, or a light board over a bed mattress. Sharp rhythmical force applied with the heel of the hand at the lower end of the sternum compresses the heart between the pliable anterior chest wall and the stable posterior thorax. The dangers inherent in this technique are from fractures of the ribs and damage to underlying viscera. These disadvantages are more than offset by the simplicity and speed with which a person with minimal training can re-establish and maintain circulation.

2 *Open chest technique* This method involves direct exposure of the heart through a left chest incision. The apex of the heart is grasped in the full hand and compressed from below upwards at a steady rate of about sixty times per minute. This method is most

feasible when the chest is already open, or when a person trained in rapid thoracotomy is immediately available.

The adequacy of circulation by either method is verified by a palpable pulse, a blood pressure over 80 mm Hg, and a small pupil. Compression ('massage') is continued until the heart is able to maintain adequate circulation by its own action.

It must be emphasized that massage with an effective perfusion is essential whether the failure of output is due to asystole or to ventricular fibrillation. Once adequate artificial perfusion has been established, the electrocardiogram becomes important to determine whether ventricular fibrillation is present. If fibrillation is present, and the heart has been effectively re-perfused with oxygenated blood, electrical defibrillation may be attempted.

The electrical current can be applied directly to the heart or by a large current through the chest wall, depending on the approach used for cardiac massage. A high current of short duration from a direct current source is preferable. Repeated applications may be necessary but only after the myocardium has been well perfused in the interval by further massage.

Drug therapy Pharmacological agents are valuable to correct tissue acidosis, to provide an inotropic boost to a flagging myocardium, or to stabilize an excessively irritable ventricle.

If, following a period of cardiac massage, spontaneous heart action is not restored and the heart is in asystole, the following steps may be taken while massage is continued:

1 Intracardiac or intravenous injection of 10 per cent calcium chloride (2–10 ml).

2 Direct or intravenous injection of adrenaline (0.2 ml 1/1000) or isoproterenol (isuprel) 1 mg/500 ml given in a drip.

3 If the asystolic heart does not respond to drug therapy, pacemaker wires can be inserted into the myocardium and electrical pacing begun.

If the heart is finely fibrillating and unresponsive to direct current shock, inotropic catecholamines (adrenaline or isuprel) may convert a fine fibrillation to a coarse type making the heart more amenable to electrical defibrillation.

Asystole may follow electrical defibrillation but continued massage often restores a spontaneous beat or, failing this, the sequence of drug therapy outlined above may be followed.

Recurring episodes of ventricular fibrillation require stabilization of the irritable cardiac membrane. Intravenous lidocaine (Xylocaine) in a 1 mg/kg bolus or a 1 mg/ml infusion is an effective membrane stabilizer and can suppress irritability sufficiently to allow effective electrical defibrillation. Intravenous lidocaine is also useful in controlling premature ventricular contractions or ventricular tachycardia.

A degree of tissue hypoxia with metabolic acidosis is inevitable in the low perfusion states that may exist before, during and after cardiac arrest. This acidosis is a further potent depressant to the heart and circulation, but can be well compensated by active pulmonary ventilation and the infusion of sodium bicarbonate buffer.

The sequelae of cardiac arrest may involve many viscera but are most significant in the brain. Any cerebral damage may be increased by reactive brain oedema which will strangle the cerebral blood flow. The onset and extent of oedema may be controlled by cerebral hypothermia, corticosteroids, or dehydration with mannitol. Continued vigilance is necessary for the delayed signs of other visceral damage or recurrence of circulatory arrest.

Resuscitation in Hypovolaemic Shock
The circulation adapts to acute loss of blood volume by a strong reflex sympathetic response, the clinical signs of which are a rapid, thready pulse, sweating, and pallor of the skin. The physiological responses are a contracted venous container to maintain venous return and arterial constriction to support the blood pressure and shift blood flow from the non-vital viscera to the heart and brain. Loss of about ten per cent of the total blood volume can be completely compensated in this manner. Further blood loss causes first a reduction in cardiac output and then hypotension. Reflex compensation is valuable but for the short term only. On a prolonged basis it becomes pathological and demands volume replacement to restore normal tissue perfusion.

Prolonged adaptation for hypovolaemia leads to visceral deterioration and autolysis with an eventual widespread loss of peripheral resistance and pooling of blood. Severe hypotension and myocardial failure soon follow. The shock is now progressive and may become irreversible. The improper use of vasopressors or an increase in the natural sympathetic amines by certain anaesthetics will speed the deterioration.

In haemorrhagic shock the keystone of treatment is restoration of blood volume to limit the stress of reflex compensation. Successful replacement therapy is tuned to the response of the patient. In most instances, stable pulse and arterial pressure without signs of sympathetic compensation signify harmony. The tuning is not so simple when cardiac disease, prolonged shock, or continued blood loss with massive replacement are present and broader contact is required to estimate the response, or lack of response, to blood transfusion. Continuous monitoring of the central venous pressure provides a convenient measure of the ability of the heart to respond to the increased load of transfusion.

The aim of treatment is to restore blood pressure by transfusion, while keeping the central venous pressure low. This relationship is more basic and valuable than blood volume determinations. Increasing central venous pressure with a poor response of arterial pressure indicates failure of the pump and points to the need for treatment other than pure volume replacement.

Myocardial depression is a frequent partner of shock during anaesthesia and accentuates the hypotension and reduced cardiac output. This cardiac failure may be from pre-existing heart disease or the influence of anaesthesia, but is more frequently a complication of shock and its treatment. Prolonged hypotension with low coronary perfusion directly limits the reserve of the heart, while poor peripheral blood flow leads to an excess accumulation of acid metabolites furthering circulatory depression.

The rapid transfusion of large quantities of blood adds other factors which may compromise cardiac function. Stored bank blood is cold, with an acid pH, and has a high potassium and low calcium content. Each of these abnormalities may weaken the heart, and each requires identification and correction by the anaesthetist.

The hazards of large volume transfusions can be greatly reduced by warming the blood to body temperature immediately before transfusion. Low serum ionized calcium, which may follow rapid excessive citrate infusion, will weaken the heart. It may be reversed by calcium gluconate if the diagnosis is supported by the electro-cardiogram. A degree of metabolic acidosis is inevitable from both the low perfusion of shock and the blood replacement. Correction of this acidosis requires both buffering with sodium bicarbonate and the guarantee of adequate respiratory compensation. A failing heart with auricular fibrillation or persistent tachycardia suggests the use of digitalis to improve myocardial function.

SUMMARY

A patient's ability to survive trauma and surgery is greatly de-pendent on the ability of the cardiocirculation system to adjust and sustain adequate delivery of oxygen to the tissues. Anaesthesia un-avoidably dampens the range of physiological adjustments possible, making proper homeostasis more difficult. The anaesthetist is as much concerned with monitoring, guarding, and assisting nature to regain control as he is in maintaining the anaesthetic state.

REFERENCES

KEATS, A.S. (editor) Symposium on Cardiology and Anesthesiology. Anesthe-siology, *33*, no. 2, (1970)

PRICE, H.L. Circulation During Anesthesia and Operation. Springfield, Ill.: Charles C. Thomas, 1967

PRICE, H.L. & COHEN, P.J. (editors). Effects of Anesthetics on the Circulation. Springfield, Ill.: Charles C. Thomas, 1964

THAL, A.P. (editor). SHOCK: A Physiological Basis for Treatment. Chicago: Year Book Medical Publisher, Inc., 1971

J.M.R. CAMPBELL

10
Fluid and electrolyte balance

A healthy person, able to take a full diet, maintains a normal fluid and electrolyte balance; that is, the amount of fluid and electrolytes taken as food and drink exactly balances the amount lost from the body, and thus the body content of them remains nearly constant.

During an operation and for varying periods following the operation, intake by mouth may not be possible and abnormal fluid losses may occur from the body, so that abnormalities of body water and electrolyte content may develop. It is then necessary to give the patient the correct amount and type of fluid, usually intravenously, to prevent the abnormalities developing or to correct any that have occurred.

NORMAL INTAKE AND OUTPUT OF WATER
AND ELECTROLYTES FROM THE BODY

In an adult the following intake and output of fluid and electrolytes normally occurs.

1 *Water*
Loss of water from the body occurs by various routes:

a Skin and Lungs A total output of 1000 to 1500 cc of water occurs each 24 hours from the skin and lungs. This loss is obligatory, always occurring even if the body is dehydrated. It occurs without visible sweating. There is no loss of electrolyte associated with this water loss.

If there is sweating a loss of 1000 to 3000 cc of water in 24 hours may easily occur and there will be some loss of electrolyte with this fluid loss.

b Kidneys The amount of water the kidney requires to excrete waste metabolites depends on the amount of metabolites and the efficiency of the kidney in concentrating urine. Five hundred cc each 24 hours is the minimum volume that must be excreted if azotaemia is not to occur. Usually 1000 to 1500 cc is excreted each 24 hours, as the maximum concentration of urine is not produced.

c Bowel Normally less than 100 cc of water is excreted through the bowel in 24 hours.

A total, then, of 2000 to 3000 ml of water is usually lost daily from the body, and there is a similar intake to maintain constant body content. Normally this amount is always taken, because loss of water produces the sensation of thirst.

2 *Sodium*
The body intake of sodium, as sodium chloride ('salt') varies greatly in amount depending on diet. Normally 1 to 2 gm/24 hours of sodium chloride is an adequate amount, though 10 to 15 gm/24 hours is often taken in food.

3 *Potassium*
There is a great variation in potassium intake, depending on the diet. However, 6 gm of potassium chloride in 24 hours is an adequate usual intake.

This daily intake of fluid and of the two common electrolytes can be used as a general guide to the amounts needed during days of the operation and the postoperative period. However, marked modifications in these amounts may be required if the patient has a deficit of water or electrolytes before the operation caused, for example, by vomiting or diarrhoea; or if he suffers excessive losses during or following the operation. In addition, the distribution of water and electrolytes within the body may be markedly altered and the body's ability to control the rate of their excretion may be impaired by the effect of the anaesthetic or the operation upon the homeostatic mechanisms.

EFFECT OF ANAESTHETIC AND OPERATION

a Collection of body fluid in the 'third space' Operative trauma commonly causes oedema formation around the site of operation. This occurs in the tissues operated upon or handled. Fluid also collects in loops of bowel which develop some degree of ileus. During and following extensive operations as much as two to five litres of fluid may be sequestrated at these sites, and this fluid has an electrolyte composition almost identical with that of the plasma. This fluid cannot be absorbed as required and is lost from the normal active available water and electrolyte content of the body. Normal body water is subdivided into intra-cellular and extra-cellular water, and as this 'lost' fluid can no longer be considered to be in these two volumes or spaces, it is referred to as being in the 'third space.' The important concept to grasp is that it is for practical purposes temporarily 'lost' from the body as effectively as it would be if it was lost externally.

b Rise of anti-diuretic hormone and adreno-cortical steroid production The stress of anaesthesia and operation leads to increased secretion of anti-diuretic hormone and adreno-cortical steroids which results in diminished ability of the kidney to excrete water and sodium.

In part the increased secretion of these hormones is due to altered distribution of fluid within the body, for example into the 'third space,' and intravenous correction of these changes in fluid distribution will lead to a lesser increase in hormone production.

Intravenous Fluids for Infusion
When there is a body deficit of water without any deficit of electrolytes an intravenous infusion of 5 per cent dextrose in water should be used. Thus no electrolytes are given and yet an isotonic intravenous fluid is used which in addition supplies some 200 calories per litre.

When there is a body deficit of sodium chloride as well as water, so called 'normal saline' may be given. However, although this is an isotonic solution, it contains a slight excess of sodium and a considerable excess of chloride as compared with amounts normally present in the plasma. Therefore when 'normal saline' is infused a relative excess of electrolyte is given, which tends to produce a hyper-chloraemic metabolic acidosis. If more than one litre of water and electrolyte is required, it is preferable to give the sodium chloride in a 'balanced electrolyte' solution. In this the sodium and chloride concentrations in the fluid are close to those present in the plasma and, in addition, potassium and calcium and possibly magnesium are present. Either acetate or lactate is present as well, which, on being broken down in the body is converted to bicarbonate, thus preventing the development of metabolic acidosis. The exact composition of different balanced electrolyte solutions vary somewhat and the appropriate one can be chosen for each patient depending on the electrolyte needs. Glucose may also be found in the balanced solution, providing a source of energy.

WATER AND ELECTROLYTE THERAPY

Intravenous Therapy for a Previously Normal Patient having an Operation
Day of operation A 70 Kgm patient should be given a total of: (*a*) 2000 cc of 5 per cent dextrose in water; (*b*) 500 cc of normal saline or balanced electrolyte solutions containing 5 per cent dextrose. This regime should cover the normal requirements of water and electrolytes. When the operation has been *extensive* with considerable tissue damage and oedema formation, then in addition: (*c*) 1000 to 3000 cc of balanced electrolyte solution containing 5 per cent dextrose may be needed to replace fluid and electrolyte lost to the 'third space.' It is a matter of careful clinical judgment how much fluid should be given for this purpose, and the volume given will depend on a careful monitoring of the clinical signs of the patient, especially the pulse and blood pressure. The condition of the peripheral veins and probably also the hourly urine output and central venous pressure should be measured.

With adequate treatment neither hypotension nor tachycardia should develop and urine volume should be at least 1000 cc in the first 24 postoperative hours.

Patients who have heart disease should be monitored with special care as they are intolerant of excess sodium chloride, and may easily develop congestive failure. Probably they should be somewhat underinfused.

Each day following operation (*a*) 500 cc of balanced electrolyte solution with 5 per cent dextrose; (*b*) 2000 to 2500 cc 5 per cent dextrose in water. This volume of water allows for an adequate urine volume, and sufficient salt intake (4 gm each 24 hours).

Potassium intake will be adequate when balanced electrolyte solutions are used. It is important when potassium is being given intravenously that there be an adequate daily urine output to allow its excretion; otherwise dangerously high potassium levels may occur with a toxic effect on the myocardium.

Intravenous Therapy for Patients who have
Abnormal Losses after Operation
Abnormal losses of fluid and electrolyte are almost always from the alimentary canal, and may occur with vomiting, diarrhoea, paralytic ileus with suction of gastric and intestinal contents, or intestinal fistulae. These losses can involve a very large volume of water, with varying proportions of sodium, chloride, and potassium, depending on which part of the alimentary canal they come from. However, for clinical purposes the fluid lost can be considered a hypotonic fluid with a sodium and chloride content slightly less than that found in plasma. The losses must be accurately measured and carefully replaced intravenously, volume for volume. Depending upon which part of the alimentary canal is losing fluid, an appropriate balanced electrolyte solution should be used for the replacement.

The daily intravenous intake for these patients will now consist of the amounts required by a normal patient as outlined above and, in addition, a volume of balanced electrolyte solution equal to that lost from the alimentary tract each 24 hours.

Intravenous Therapy for Patients with Preoperative
Severe Water and Electrolyte Loss

Water and electrolyte losses should be corrected as far as possible before operation. This will reduce the mortality and morbidity of operation. Moreover, it is more difficult to correct a deficit post-operatively because of the changes in fluid balance and hormone excretion occurring at that time owing to the stress of the operation.

The first step in preoperative treatment is to determine as accurately as possible the extent of the water and/or salt deficiency. Three patterns are possible:

1 The patient may be deficient in water, but have little salt deficiency. An example would be an unconscious patient who has had no fluid intake for 36 hours and who, during this time, has continued to lose water automatically from lungs and skin.

2 The patient may have primarily a salt deficiency; an example would be a patient who has had severe vomiting or diarrhoea, but has been able to drink and absorb water.

3 The patient may have a deficiency of both water and salt in the proportion in which they are present in body fluids; this would be true of a patient with vomiting or diarrhoea who has been unable to drink water.

The term 'dehydration' is often used to describe any of the above patterns of loss, but an attempt should always be made to differentiate between them, as the treatment varies.

EXTENT AND TYPE OF DEFICIENCY

This is often difficult to estimate with any degree of accuracy, for there is no single or simple test that will given the answer. One must consider the following:

1 *History* Information should be obtained, where possible, of both the type and extent of losses, and of the fluid intake during the past 24 hours.

2 *Physical Examination* Careful examination of the patient, with particular attention to: (*a*) the general condition of the patient,

especially the mental state, presence or absence of thirst and presence or absence of anorexia or nausea; (*b*) the state of turgor of the skin and moisture of the mucous membranes; (*c*) the state of the cardiovascular system, paying particular attention to the superficial veins, the temperature of the extremities, and the pulse and blood pressure.

3 *Laboratory Tests* (*a*) Urine should be examined for specific gravity, amount of chloride present, and the hourly urine volume excreted. (*b*) The haemoglobin and plasma protein concentration, serum electrolytes and blood urea should be estimated.

The results of the tests depend on the fact that the general disturbance produced by a water deficiency alone differs from the disturbance produced when the main and primary deficit is lack of salt, with only a secondary loss of water.

Water Loss Alone
The water loss is borne proportionally by both the intracellular and the extracellular compartments of the body; it produces in both a decreased volume and an increased osmolarity.

Primary Salt Loss
Sodium chloride is mostly present in the extracellular compartment, which includes the plasma. As sodium chloride is lost from the body, water is also excreted as the body attempts to maintain the normal osmolarity of the extracellular fluid. As little or no sodium chloride is lost from the intracellular compartment, the body does not lose water from there. Therefore, the water that is lost secondary to the salt loss comes largely from the extracellular compartment, including plasma. Circulatory secondary renal failure occurs earlier than when the same volume of water is lost from the body in a pure water deficiency.

For example, suppose a patient has lost 3 to 4 L of body water. This may have occurred as a pure water loss, or as a water loss secondary to a primary salt loss. The symptoms and signs shown in Table I may be expected.

Definite evidence of dehydration according to the criteria of

Table I

Clinical features	Pure water loss	Water loss secondary to salt loss
	Weakness, ill look, feverish late	Weakness, apathy, giddiness, mental confusion, stupor, anorexia, nausea and vomiting
Thirst	Intense	Not remarkable
Skin turgor	Normal or rubbery	Decreased
Pulse	Slightly raised	Rapid
Blood pressure	Normal or slightly down	Low
Cold cyanotic extremities, with collapsed veins	Slight	Marked
	LABORATORY FINDINGS	
Urine		
volume	300–500 cc/day	Unaltered till late
specific gravity	Maximal	Low to normal
chlorides	Over 5 gm/L	Under 3 gm/L
Blood		
Hbg and Hct	Increased late	Increased early
proteins	Increased late	Increased early
blood urea	High normal	Elevated early
plasma sodium	Elevated	Reduced

Table I implies a deficiency of at least 4000 cc. If there is a history of loss of fluid, but no obvious signs of dehydration, the patient is probably about 2000 cc deficient.

Treatment (*a*) If acute dehydration is due to inadequate intake, make up the deficiency with 5 per cent dextrose in water. (*b*) If acute losses have occurred from the alimentary tract, replace the loss with appropriate balanced electrolyte solution.

If dehydration has been acute in onset, the replacement can be given rapidly; that is, the estimated requirement of fluid can be given in two hours. During this period the patient should be observed for signs of overinfusion, such as crepitations at the lung bases or overdistended jugular veins. Once the estimated requirement of fluid has been given, the patient's condition should be reassessed to see if he requires more fluid. The clinical and laboratory examinations mentioned previously should be repeated and, depending on the findings, more fluid may be given.

Recording of Fluid and Electrolyte Status

Finally, it is essential in the treatment of patients requiring intra-venous fluid therapy that an accurate Fluid Balance Chart be kept from the time of operation or, ideally, for 24 hours before that time. The type and volume of all fluid given should be recorded, as should the volume and route by which fluid is lost from the body. This chart is an essential aid for the successful planning of effective therapy.

H.B.F. FAIRLEY

11
Acid-base balance

Hydrogen ion concentration ($[H^+]$) varies from tissue to tissue according to metabolic activity and differs in intracellular and extracellular fluid. Essentially, the human organism 'activates' large quantities of hydrogen ion (H^+) as a result of metabolism of carbohydrates, fats, and proteins, producing substances such as carbonic acid, acid phosphates, and sulphates – all capable of H^+ donation.

For normal physiological processes to proceed, $[H^+]$ must be maintained within relatively narrow limits. These limits are usually discussed in terms of arterial blood (i.e., rejuvenated, distal to the respiratory mechanism and before addition of further H^+ from tissues). However, this is a most indirect assessment of the various optimal $[H^+]$ levels of the different body tissues.

NORMAL RANGE OF HYDROGEN ION CONCENTRATION

A solution is neutral, from the standpoint of acid-base balance, when the hydrogen ion concentration is $1/10,000,000$ gm/L, i.e. 10^{-7} gm/L. This is referred to as a pH of 7, in the same way that a solution with a $[H^+]$ of $1/100,000,000$ gm/L (10^{-8}) is said to have a pH of 8. Figure 1 shows that this range (pH7–8) can also be quoted directly in hydrogen ion concentration units, rather than as their reciprocal. Since 10^{-9} M/L is 1 nanomole, 10^{-8} M/L

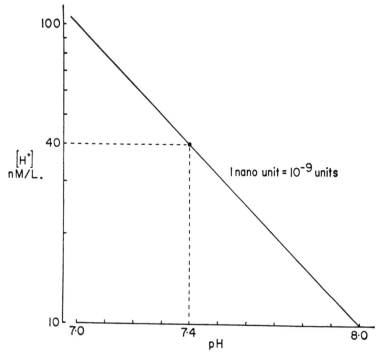

FIGURE 1

(pH 8) is 10 nanomoles, and the range pH 7–8 is the same as 100–10 nanomoles.

Normal arterial blood has a hydrogen ion concentration of between 1/22,387,200 gm/L and 1/28,184,800 gm/L, i.e., a pH between 7.35 and 7.45 (45–35 nM/L).

SOURCES OF HYDROGEN IONS AND ROUTES OF ELIMINATION

Hydrogen ions are normally present in body water but are largely undissociated and are electrically balanced by hydroxyl ions. However, various metabolic products dissociate more readily and contribute free H^+ not electrically balanced by hydroxyl ions. This rise in the [H+] is offset by three protective mechanisms: (a) buffering, (b) ventilation, (c) renal excretion. A most important point to grasp is the gross difference between the last two defences against hydrogen ion accumulation. The respiratory system excretes approximately 200 times more milliequivalents of 'acid' than the kidney in a 24-hour period. Of course, this is restricted to carbon dioxide, and most of the hydrogen ions excreted by the kidney are associated with non-volatile substances. This quantitative distinction is important, for it suggests the speed with which acidosis occurs when the respiratory mechanism fails, as opposed to when the kidneys fails, and it indicates the quantitative effectiveness of hyperventilation in the immediate management of acidosis.

ACID-BASE ABNORMALITIES IN PATIENTS
REQUIRING ANAESTHESIA

Since anaesthesia and surgery inevitably impose restrictions on normal hydrogen ion balance (see below), any pre-existing abnormality may have exaggerated implications. These may be: (a) disorders of buffering, e.g. severe anaemia, low total cation levels; (b) disorders of elimination, e.g. respiratory or renal disease; (c) excessive production of H+, e.g., when tissue oxygenation is inadequate, carbohydrate metabolism cannot be completed and excessive quantities of lactic acid are formed. This lactacidosis is common and may be most serious. It occurs in hypoxia, whether related to respiratory problems, congenital heart disease, or peripheral vascular failure. It is a usual accompaniment of 'shock' and dehydration. Ketotic acidosis is seen occasionally, caused by starvation or diabetes mellitus.

When a patient comes to the operating room with a non-respiratory acidosis due, for example, to renal failure, it is important to recognize that he will probably be spontaneously overventilating. Any depression of his central awareness of this need may then result in a dramatic accentuation of the acidosis.

Most rarely, patients may come to the operating room in alkalosis. Overventilation, in association with pneumonia or head injury, is one of the more common causes. Occasionally, untreated pyloric obstruction or prolonged naso-gastric suction may produce a significant loss of H^+ and present a problem to the anaesthetist. Alkalosis may also be due to hypokalaemia.

ACID-BASE ABNORMALITIES ARISING DURING AND AFTER ANAESTHESIA

The respiratory neurones are depressed by narcotics and by inhalation anaesthetic agents. Consequently, respiratory compensation for H^+ excess is disturbed. During anaesthesia in which spontaneous respiration is permitted, a mild accumulation of carbon dioxide is usual, and the arterial P_{CO_2} may rise to between 45 and 60 mm Hg without gross clinical manifestations.

Light anaesthesia causes no significant change in non-respiratory hydrogen ion balance. However, hypovolaemia due to blood loss may produce lactacidosis and may depress renal function. Massive transfusion will add significant quantities of acid citrate and lactic acid.

When spontaneous respiration is replaced by manual or mechanical ventilation, widely varying volumes may result, and no 'automatic' compensation for $[H^+]$ abnormality exists.

Postoperatively, the respiratory neurones usually return to normal responsiveness quite quickly but, occasionally, this is prevented by central or peripheral depression or by pain on respiration.

CONSEQUENCE OF ACID-BASE IMBALANCE

An abnormal $[H^+]$ has three practical implications: (a) It is an index of its causative pathology and of the course of the pathology. (b) It may be hazardous in itself. (c) Changes in $[H^+]$ change the dose response to many drugs. Respiratory alkalosis is common during anaesthesia and in patients receiving mechanical ventilation for respiratory failure. In most instances it is tolerated very well and, as a consequence, many anaesthetists prefer to err on the side of overventilation in situations where acid-base monitoring is not immediately available. However, three possible consequences of respiratory alkalosis should be mentioned. (a) Under anaesthesia, cardiac output varies directly with arterial carbon dioxide tension. (b) An acute increase in ventilation of patients with cardiac disease may produce a change in cardiac rhythm. The mechanism is uncertain but probably relates to an acute change in intracellular/extracellular distribution of potassium ions. In digitalized patients with marginally low potassium levels, this may be particularly hazardous. (c) Respiratory alkalosis produces cerebral vasoconstriction, but it is questionable whether it is ever sufficient to produce permanent cerebral damage. Indeed, there are those who advocate this as a means of redistributing flow from normal to insufficient (and therefore maximally dilated and non-responsive) areas – the so-called Robin Hood effect. High [H$^+$], whether produced by respiratory or non-respiratory causes, can be extremely serious. Among its harmful effects are central nervous system depression leading to coma, cardiovascular depression leading to hypotension or even to cardiac arrest, and depression of activity of such agents as digitalis and catecholamines.

EVALUATION OF ACID-BASE BALANCE

Clinically, acid-base balance is extremely difficult to evaluate other than by assumptions based on aetiologies. There is no satisfactory alternative to blood analysis. Preferably, arterial blood should be drawn anaerobically in a heparinized syringe and analysed immediately. With careful techniques, capillary or venous blood from the back of a warmed hand may be used on the assumption that this will provide results similar to those from arterial blood. However, it is usually helpful to know the Pa$_{O_2}$ at the same time, in which case arterial blood is almost essential.

It is useful to consider overall acid-base status first, then to separate this into respiratory and non-respiratory components.

Overall Status

pH values between 7.35 and 7.45 are normal, but a value in this range does not indicate whether both respiratory and non-respiratory components are normal. If one is abnormal, a complementary abnormality in the other may produce a normal [H$^+$]. As a rule of thumb, values below pH 7.3 are serious; with values below pH 7.15, patients are usually comatose and in immediate danger of death. Values below pH 7 (to pH 6.7) are only seen in association with the grossest abnormalities (e.g. during cardiac massage) and are associated with an extremely high mortality.

Respiratory component Arterial carbon dioxide tension (Pa_{CO_2}) is mentioned in Chapter 8, Respiration and Anaesthesia. Normal values are 38–42 mm Hg. In association with pH values, Pa_{CO_2} determination offers the only absolute measure of ventilation. For example, a pH of 7.2 and a Pa_{CO_2} of 75 would indicate acute respiratory acidosis. A pH of 7.6 and a Pa_{CO_2} of 20 would indicate acute respiratory alkalosis. If these states of acute respiratory change were maintained over a period of hours and days, an adjustment of pH towards normal would occur by a process of renal excretion or retention of H^+. As this occurred the pH values illustrated above might change serially towards normal. It would be unusual for the compensation to be complete, however.

Non-respiratory status A more difficult problem is to evaluate that portion of the $[H^+]$, whether primary or secondary, which is not related to respiratory change. This is commonly done in one of four ways.

1 From pH and Pa_{CO_2} values alone. Acidosis not related to CO_2 retention (e.g. pH 7.2, Pa_{CO_2} 35 mm Hg) must be non-respiratory in origin. The pH and Pa_{CO_2} give an index of the extent of respiratory compensation for the non-respiratory disorder, expressed in the pH as the algebraic sum of the two. The other methods, giving absolute values for the non-respiratory component, are more useful.

2 Blood buffer base: quantitating all the anions available for buffering. Four main buffer pairs exist in blood: $HCO_3^-/H \cdot HCO_3$; $Pr^-/H \cdot Pr$; $HPO_4^-/H \cdot HPO_4$; $Hgb^-/H \cdot Hgb$. The first two pairs are mainly in the plasma, while the latter two pairs are in the red cells and are related in quantity to the haemoglobin level. This total buffer anion is the blood buffer base and has a normal value, in mEq/L, of $40.8 + 0.36 \times Hgb$ (in gm %), or approximately 45 mEq/L, when Pa_{CO_2} is 40 mm Hg.

3 Base excess: This involves the concept that, when a blood sample

is maintained at 37° C and P_{CO_2} 40, any deviation of pH from normal must be due to non-respiratory factors. This may be quantitated as the amount of acid or base necessary to restore pH to 7.4. Results are expressed as mEq/L above or below 0. Alkalosis is referred to as positive base excess and acidosis as negative base excess.

This most useful means of obtaining (usually from a nomogram) a value in mEq/L for the magnitude of any non-respiratory acid-base disorder is widely used. However, it has been rightly criticized because it involves data derived *in vitro* from a blood sample. This prevents any consideration of whole body buffering capacity, i.e. the "bicarbonate space" involves not only the efficient buffering of blood and the equally high HCO_3^- levels in extracellular fluid, but also the intracellular fluid. Detractors claim that calculation of, say, the necessary dose of sodium bicarbonate to correct a non-respiratory acidosis, from a base excess value multiplied by an estimated whole body bicarbonate space, will frequently be misleading. However, in practice (see TREATMENT below), it is possible to put base excess values to good use.

Normal limits for base excess are ±3 mEq/L.

4 Bicarbonate As the carbon dioxide tension of blood changes there is an immediate change in $[HCO_3^-]$ in the same direction. When the carbon dioxide tension is returned to normal, $[HCO_3^-]$ also returns. Any deviation of $[HCO_3^-]$ from 24 mEq/L at 37° C and P_{CO_2} 40 (standard bicarbonate) indicates non-respiratory change. If $[HCO_3^-]$ values are available at a P_{CO_2} level other than 40, it is necessary to know the normal under these circumstances. Whole body CO_2 titrations have now been performed in man and 95 per cent confidence limits for $[HCO_3^-]$ defined.

It is noteworthy that, at high P_{CO_2} levels (i.e. above 70 mm Hg), the rise in $[HCO_3^-]$ for each increment of P_{CO_2} is not as great at lower values.

There is a body of opinion to the effect that non-respiratory acid-base imbalance is best assessed by $[HCO_3^-]$ level derived from pH and P_{CO_2} values. When the latter are plotted on a graphic representation of the Henderson–Hasselbach equation (with isopleths for the third variable) the $[HCO_3^-]$ can be derived. If whole body titration confidence limits for [HCO_3^-] are plotted on the diagram, at all levels of P_{CO_2}, [HCO_3^-] deviation from normal can be read off in mEq/L. There is probably general agreement that this is a highly accurate method of evaluation and that, short of a whole body titration curve for the particular patient involved, this represents the closest one can come to the truth.

In the author's opinion, there is little to choose in practice and local custom will probably dictate the method of choice. Each involves the measurement of pH and P_{CO_2} and an extrapolation to whole body circumstances, through an estimate of the magnitude of the non-respiratory disturbance and of the patient's HCO_3^-.

TREATMENT

Primary treatment for all acid-base balance disturbances must lie in the correction of aetiological factors, and in most instances this is all that is required. When pH is seriously deranged, especially in the direction of acidosis, 'symptomatic' treatment may be indicated. Increased ventilation may be most useful and will be the definitive treatment for acute respiratory acidosis. When non-respiratory acidosis is present, and especially when pH is below 7.2, sodium bicarbonate or THAM may be given intravenously. As a practical rule of thumb, the total extracellular fluid volume may be calculated (20 per cent of body weight in kilograms) and the theoretical H^+ excess calculated (from blood buffer base deficit, negative base excess, or drop in bicarbonate). Half this calculated quantity is then given as milliequivalents of sodium bicarbonate or THAM. Further blood values are then obtained and the procedure repeated. The actual H^+ excess of the whole organism will be considerably greater than that calculated for an extracellular space of 20 per cent of body weight. For whole body calculations, various figures up to 50 per cent of body weight have been suggested, factors of 0.3–0.4 being commonly used.

An important consideration in the assessment and management of acid-base disturbance is the different rates at which carbon dioxide and HCO_3^- pass between CSF and blood. HCO_3^- passes extremely slowly and, as a consequence, any change produced in blood will not be mimicked immediately in CSF. Two important clinical consequences are mentioned as examples: First, the patient with chronic CO_2 retention and consequent high $[HCO_3^-]$ in blood and cerebro-spinal fluid (CSF), who develops an additional acute respiratory acidosis. If his Pa_{CO_2} is rapidly returned to normal, a profound CSF alkalosis and cerebral vasoconstriction result and, on occasion, an encephalopathy may follow. The only solution is to reduce the Pa_{CO_2} of such patients slowly over a period of hours. Another example is the patient who is overventilating because of chronic renal acidosis. He is to be anaesthetized and it is decided to correct his acidosis with $NaHCO_3$. He does not stop hyperventilating even though his non-respiratory acidosis is reversed in blood. He now has marked respiratory alkalosis. However, his CSF acid-base balance is probably not greatly altered since little of the $NaHCO_3$ has reached the CSF. Under anaesthesia, there is then the difficult problem of knowing at what level to maintain ventilation.

Permeability of the blood-brain barrier to CO_2 and HCO_3^- (as exemplified by blood/CSF differences) is obviously important in the central control of respiration and circulation. While gross discrepanices must obviously be corrected, these examples are included to discourage an over-zealous approach to acid-base balance manipulation.

A final factor which should be mentioned is that of time in relation to clinical course. Frequently, blood data for acid-base status is obtained during the unsteady state both from the respiratory and non-respiratory standpoint. Before responding to the data, one should consider the direction of the clinical course in the interval. Indeed, a second blood sample may then provide very valuable information as to progress, and presence or lack of urgency.

C.C. STODDARD AND R.A. GORDON

12
Complications of anaesthesia

As surgery is being offered to more seriously ill patients and has invaded all the more sacred areas of the body such as the brain, heart, and lungs, complications naturally increase and take on a more serious nature.

Compensating for this, however, is the increased knowledge that has been gained during recent years through research, study, new drugs, and new anaesthetic agents and techniques. Skilled anaesthetists stress the prevention of complications, diagnose them as soon as they occur, and institute early treatment.

In this chapter the more serious complications will be reviewed in some detail while other less serious ones will be briefly discussed. Further references are given in the bibliography at the end of the chapter.

The physical condition of the patient prior to induction of anaesthesia is of utmost importance in anticipating possible complications. Heart disease, congenital and acquired, arterio-sclerosis, extreme youth and old age, debility, trauma and shock, metabolic disease, and lung disease enhance the possibility of complications resulting from anaesthesia.

RESPIRATORY COMPLICATIONS

Respiratory obstruction of any sort creates physiological changes that will soon injure the brain, heart, liver, and kidneys. Obstruction should never be allowed to persist but should be immediately diagnosed and corrected. A prime requisite for a good anaesthetic is a clear unobstructed airway at all times. A clear airway allows oxygenation of the blood in the lungs and exhalation of carbon dioxide in the expired air.

Upper Respiratory Obstruction
The tongue may fall back against the posterior pharyngeal wall and obstruct the flow of air or gases to the trachea. In most patients all that will be necessary to correct this situation is to bring the angle of the jaw forward with the hand, thereby raising the tongue. In edentulous old people it may also be necessary to pull the tongue forward manually and insert an oropharyngeal airway. If the airway is placed in the pharynx with the patient in a very light stage of anaesthesia, coughing or laryngeal spasm may result.

If this method fails, a muscle relaxant should be given intravenously and a tracheal tube inserted. Occasionally patients may arrive in the operating theatre with their false teeth in place. During the anaesthetic the denture may become dislodged and create a complete obstruction above the vocal cords. It is therefore wise to examine every patient's mouth for dentures and to remove them. A similar problem may arise from loose teeth or bridges which become dislodged with various manipulations. Treatment is to remove such objects from the pharynx with forceps.

Malformations of the jaws, tongue, or trachea, and enlarged thyroid pressing on the trachea, can easily be recognized preoperatively, and special steps can be taken to reduce the hazard of anaesthesia. For example, nasal intubation, intubation after topical anaesthesia with the patient awake, or tracheotomy prior to induction of general anaesthesia may have to be considered.

Mucus and saliva may accumulate in the pharynx, particularly during induction of light anaesthesia and should be immediately removed by suction. Suctioning should not be too vigorous or prolonged as the delicate tissues in the pharynx and around the cords may be traumatized. The incidence of trauma may be reduced by occluding the suction catheter by pressure with the fingers and then releasing the pressure for a few seconds at a time.

Laryngeal spasm The larynx is primarily a valve designed to prevent foreign matter from entering the air passages. The vocal cords abduct during inspiration and adduct during expiration. The muscles are amazingly strong. The natural reaction of the larynx to stimulation by drugs and foreign bodies is to go into spasm in adduction, thus preventing anything from entering the air passages. Laryngeal spasm may occur in the early stages of anaesthesia, especially when one uses an irritating anaesthetic agent such as ether.

Some patients have excessive bronchial secretions which may appear after a sudden cough and create laryngospasm. If there has been some regurgitation of stomach contents into the pharynx, laryngospasm will occur and remain until the irritant is removed. Intravenous induction of anaesthesia may cause coughing and laryngospasm, especially in patients with chronic bronchitis or asthma; these agents seem to create hyperactivity of the reflexes in the pharynx and larynx, resulting in spasm. Stimulation from the operative site, especially in the abdomen and chest while the patient is under light general anaesthesia, may also initiate laryngospasm. Mucus or vomitus should be aspirated immediately, but the larynx should not be irritated with the suction catheter. An adequate dose of atropine should be given one-half to three-quarters of an hour preoperatively, and in emergency or out-patient cases it should be given intravenously. If the patient has asthma or chronic bronchitis, adequate therapy for these conditions should be given before the patient appears for an anaesthetic. Adequate preoperative sedation plus cortisone therapy will be of great value.

If laryngeal spasm occurs, discontinue the anaesthetic; give oxygen only. Stop the operation and apply steady pressure on the re-breathing bag of the gas machine. If the spasm persists then succinylcholine must be given intravenously and a tracheal tube inserted. Adequate ventilation can then be accomplished.

Oedema of the larynx may be due to trauma associated with tracheal intubation; it may result from using too large a tube, or from excessive inflation of its cuff. Allergic reaction to the rubber tube or lubricant or topical anaesthetic may cause laryngeal oedema. Recent or latent infection will predispose a patient to this complication.

Tracheal intubation should be done with the utmost gentleness. Tracheal tubes should be inserted far enough to ensure that the cuff is beyond the vocal cords. Patients who have had recent infections (e.g. laryngitis) should not have a tracheal intubation unless it is absolutely necessary.

Antiallergic drugs may help in treatment. Steam inhalations will be of some value if stridor develops postoperatively.

Lower Respiratory Obstruction

Bronchospasm The bronchial muscles are supplied by the sympathetic and parasympathetic nervous systems. The sympathetic dilates the bronchi, constricts the bronchial arteries, and reduces or stops secretions, while the parasympathetic has the opposite effect.

Bronchospasm is likely to occur when the vagus is stimulated by histamine release from intravenous anaesthetics, cyclopropane, or d-tubocurare. The sensitivity of the respiratory tract increases from above downward and is greatest at the carina. The propensity to these reflexes varies with individuals and is increased in nervous young patients, in those in great pain and in those suffering from asthma, chronic bronchitis, or other lung disease. It is decreased in the aged and very ill.

Usually there is a history of chronic lung disease. Often bronchospasm occurs after the patient has been intubated. There is difficulty in inflating the lungs and in maintaining oxygenation, because of the small tidal exchange and prolonged forceful expiration, often with 'bucking.' In extreme cases one cannot inflate the lungs at all and there may be no return of air from the lungs, owing to air trapping. On auscultation the breath sounds are reduced and musical; high-pitched rhonchi are heard throughout the chest. Suction does not reveal any sputum unless it has been the initiating cause.

Avoid the use of thiopentone and d-tubocurare if there is a history of chronic lung disease or asthma. Prepare the patient well beforehand with therapy suitable to the situation, such as antibiotics, antihistamines (e.g. promethazine), cortisone, bronchodilators (e.g. atropine, isoprenoline). The patient should be well anaesthetized before manipulations such as intubation and surgery are attempted.

When bronchospasm occurs, aerate the lungs as well as possible with oxygen; suction sputum if present but do not aspirate too often, as this may increase the anoxia and cause cardiac arrest. Atropine 0.6 mg intravenously may help. Aminophyllin and cortisone intravenously are useful drugs, particularly if the patient is asthmatic. Muscle relaxants such as succinylcholine should be given to improve the airway and relax the muscles of respiration. Deflating the cuff of the tracheal tube may help, but it would be unwise to remove the tube even if bronchospasm has occurred immediately after insertion.

Aspiration of gastric contents Aspiration of gastric contents is considered one of the most serious complications that may confront the anaesthetist in the induction period, during the operative phase, and in the postanaesthetic period. It has been calculated that 2 per cent of all maternal deaths in the United States are directly due to aspiration of vomitus.

The results of aspiration of stomach contents vary with the nature of the material aspirated. The presence of solid food material in the bronchial tree results in atelectasis, mediastinal shift, cyanosis, dyspnoea, and tachycardia which clear after the obstruction is removed. Aspiration of acid fluid from the stomach produces dyspnoea, cyanosis, tachycardia, bronchospasm, and diffusely scattered densities in the X-ray; these patients tend to go on to cardiac failure and pulmonary oedema, followed by early death or, in survivors, signs of clinical improvement in 24 to 48 hours. If both solids and liquids are aspirated the signs and symptoms will be a mixture of those described above.

When vomitus has been aspirated examination of the lungs reveals rales and rhonchi in some areas, no aeration in others. Inflation of the lungs is difficult. If aspiration occurs during the induction period it may be detected by audible bubbling or laryngospasm, but if anaesthesia has been established there may be silent regurgitation. Silent regurgitation may be caused by distension of the stomach by air during the ventilation of an apnoeic patient.

Prevention of aspiration must be emphasized. Special attention must be paid to accident cases, since in these patients the stomach will rarely be empty, even though the accident has occurred six to eight hours prior to the anaesthetic. Gastric peristalsis usually stops at the time of a severe accident. Obstetrical patients are often encouraged to swallow fluids up to the time of delivery. It is difficult to be sure that the stomach of a child is empty. Except for properly prepared elective cases, all patients should be treated as having full stomachs. Drainage of the stomach through a stomach tube prior to induction reduces the danger of gastric reflux, but does not remove the hazard.

Special methods of induction have been advocated to reduce the hazard of regurgitation and vomiting. No matter what method is used the anaesthetist must assure himself beforehand that the suction equipment is adequate, that the laryngoscope is in good working order, and that the cuffs on tracheal tubes have been checked for leaks.

Some anaesthetists advocate placing the patient on the left side with the head down so that regurgitated gastric contents will run out of the mouth. Induction is then accomplished with an intravenous barbiturate such as thiopentone, relaxation with succinylcholine, and rapid intubation of the trachea using a cuffed tube. Others recommend the same type of induction with the patient in the usual supine position. Induction with the patient tilted into a semi-sitting or head-up position has been advocated to prevent the passive reflux of fluid from the stomach, and occlusion of the oesophagus by having an assistant press firmly backwards on the cricoid cartilage has been recommended. Other anaesthetists believe that a cuffed tube should be inserted into the trachea of the conscious patient under topical anaesthesia whenever serious danger of regurgitation exists. Certainly inflation of the stomach should be avoided by oxygenating the patient prior to induction, rather than by ventilation after induction.

When vomiting or regurgitation is recognized, treatment must be instituted immediately. Solid material must be scooped out of the mouth and pharynx promptly with fingers or forceps, and the pharynx must be cleared of all fluid by suction. If the jaws are clenched due to light anaesthesia, suction through the nose should be employed, the patient should be put into a steep Trendelenburg position, and the mouth should be forced open by a mouth gag. If it is possible to clear the upper airway in this fashion, the patient should be re-oxygenated and the trachea should then be intubated with a cuffed tube under relaxation produced by a short-acting muscle relaxant. It must be recognized, however, that the patient's survival depends on immediate control of the airway, and in the face of difficulty in clearing the material from the pharynx a short-acting muscle relaxant should be given promptly to permit immediate intubation. With the tracheal tube in place the patient should be ventilated with oxygen, and the trachea and bronchi should be suctioned repeatedly to remove fluid, the patient being re-oxygenated after each brief interval of suction.

Some anaesthetists recommend bronchial lavage with sterile normal saline to lessen the degree of bronchospasm and pulmonary oedema. This is done by injecting 5 to 10 cc of sterile normal saline into the tracheal tube, followed immediately by endotracheal and endobronchial suction and re-oxygenation. The manoeuvre is repeated until the aspirated fluid is clear. This treatment is regarded as controversial, and many feel that it serves only to force the aspirated material further into the lungs.

Aminophyllin or an antihistamine (e.g. pyribenzamine) should be given intravenously to combat bronchospasm, and may have to be repeated several times. Hydrocortisone should be given intravenously at once in doses of 400 to 500 mg to counteract inflammatory reaction and bronchospasm. Pulmonary oedema may be helped by positive pressure breathing. Antibiotics are given to combat infection. Bronchoscopy may be required to remove solid matter or to encourage re-expansion of atelectatic areas. The tracheal tube should not be removed until the patient is fully awake, with active laryngeal reflexes.

If marked respiratory distress persists, the tracheal tube should be kept in place or a tracheotomy may be required. Tracheotomy is the method of choice if the patient is likely to require respiratory assistance for longer than 24 hours. If respiration is inadequate, a respirator should be used to control or assist respiration. The patient must be watched most carefully during the first 48 hours to assess general condition and to diagnose and treat pulmonary complications.

Complications of Tracheal Intubation

Tracheal intubation is accepted practice for general anaesthesia in patients requiring operations on the head and neck, chest, upper abdomen, and in the prone position, as well as in other selected cases. There are many complications associated with intubation.

1 *Insertion of tube into right main bronchus* The right bronchus forms an obtuse angle with the trachea while the angle formed by the left main bronchus is more acute. If the tracheal tube is inserted beyond the carina, it will enter the right main bronchus. If this is undetected, the patient will breath with the right lung, while the other will collapse over a period of time. Unilateral movement of the chest and absence of breath sounds on the left side will confirm the diagnosis. The tube should be withdrawn until breath sounds are heard over the left lung.

2 *Kinking of the tube* Tracheal tubes which are too long or too soft may become obstructed by kinking either inside the oral cavity or outside the mouth. The signs of respiratory obstruction are increased respiratory effort, indrawing of the chest wall and supracostal spaces, difficulty in ventilating the patient by compressing the reservoir bag. These will be followed rapidly by signs of anoxia and accumulation of CO_2. Tubes must be firm and cut to a proper length, so that the metal connector rests between the lips.

3 *Insertion of tube into the oesophagus* Accidental intubation of the oesophagus can occur whenever there is difficulty in exposing the cords, and will result in distension of the stomach. Short sharp pressure on the chest produces a characteristic puff of air after tracheal intubation, which may be replaced by a characteristic sucking sound if the tube is in the oesophagus. If this situation is not recognized, the stomach will gradually become distended with gas,

forcing the diaphragm up and collapsing the lungs. The patient rapidly becomes cyanosed and cardiac arrest may occur unless corrective measures are instituted immediately. The tube should be removed, the lungs inflated with oxygen, and the tube then reinserted in the proper position. It may be necessary to introduce a stomach tube to deflate the stomach.

4 *Traumatic complications of intubation* Traumatic complications may usually be avoided by gentleness and good judgment. The lips or tongue may be caught between the teeth and the blade of the laryngoscope causing severe bruises or cuts. Teeth may be chipped, loosened, or dislodged. Lacerations or haemorrhage of the pharyngeal mucous membranes may be produced by the blade of the laryngoscope under poor vision, nasal haemorrhage may be produced by forceful insertion of the nasal tube, and adenoid tissue may be dislodged, especially in children. Submucous haemorrhage in the region of the false vocal cords may be produced by traumatic intubation. Failure to anchor the tracheal tube properly may lead to displacement of the tube into the pharynx or the bronchus. Coughing or bucking on the tube may cause irritation to the trachea and the cords. Vagal reflexes causing cardiac irregularities or cardiac arrest may occur, especially under light anaesthesia. Intubation may be followed by oedema of the larynx, tracheitis, and ulceration or granuloma of the vocal cords.

Pneumothorax

Pneumothorax may occur in the course of anaesthesia or surgery in many ways. High pressures from a gas machine directed into the lungs may rupture the alveoli, causing haemorrhage and dissection of air into the interstitial tissues. This in turn may rupture into the pleural cavity or dissect back into the mediastinum. Air in the mediastinum under pressure may rupture retroperitoneally, or, after rupture of the mediastinal pleura, may rupture into the pleural cavity. One cannot determine the pressure required to rupture alveoli, but it has been estimated that pressures of 18 to 24 mm Hg are within safe limits.

The common causes of pneumothorax during anaesthesia are

(a) high inflation pressures, sometimes due to faulty valves in the anaesthetic machine; (b) faulty placement of needles for regional anaesthesia, e.g., brachial plexus, intercostal and thoracic sympathetic blocks; (c) inadvertently induced surgical pneumothoraces in dissections of the neck and tracheotomy, in stellate ganglioectomy, in thoracotomy, in operations on the kidneys and adrenal glands, during subclavian and carotid angiography, and through tears of the oesophagus from endoscopy.

When a pneumothorax occurs, a conscious patient may complain of mild pain in the chest or shoulder and mild dyspnoea which increases with moving about. If a tension pneumothorax occurs, these symptoms will progress to pronounced dyspnoea, cyanosis, tachycardia, and respiratory obstruction followed by cardiovascular collapse. In the patient under anaesthesia there may be tachycardia and cyanosis, difficulty in ventilation, hypotension, and cardiac arrest. Tension pneumothorax is more likely to occur when positive pressure ventilation is being used. Whenever there is respiratory and circulatory embarrassment, pneumothorax should be suspected. The diagnosis may be confirmed by X-ray, but the urgency of the situation seldom allows this. On auscultation there will be no air entry on the affected side of the chest if the lung is completely collapsed. Percussion gives a resonant note, but shift of the trachea to the opposite side is perhaps the most useful sign to the anaesthetist.

Treatment may be urgent, and requires aspiration of the air from the pleural space and continuous suction or water-sealed drainage of the chest. At the same time, positive pressure should be applied to the airway to assist in re-expansion of the lung.

Atelectasis

Atelectasis or collapse of a lung, both lungs, or part of a lung may occur during anaesthesia or in the postoperative period. Acute collapse is frequently not associated with evidence of obstruction or congestion of the bronchi usually found when the onset is gradual. It has been suggested that respiratory depression, rapid absorption of gases from the alveoli, and bronchospasm secondary to vagus nerve reflexes may be the causative factors. Churchill-Davidson has suggested that spasm of the bronchial musculature not only would reduce the size of the lumen but also might be sufficient to cause further obstruction by impeding the venous return while still allowing arterial blood to be pumped into the capillary plexus. This would result in oedema of the bronchial or mucous membrane, making rapid collapse possible.

Atelectasis may be caused by mucous plugs in the bronchus or bronchi or by a foreign body in the trachea, examples being broken teeth, aspirated gastric contents, or a tracheal tube placed in the right bronchus.

Atelectasis may go unrecognized in the unconscious patient who is being well ventilated. Signs of hypoxia, tachycardia, or deficient breathing should lead one to examine the chest. Such examination will reveal absence of air entry into the affected lobe or lobes. The patient may or may not be cyanotic, depending on the degree of collapse. Tachypnoea is a universal finding, the temperature is elevated, and the mediastinum shifted to the affected side (tracheal shift).

Treatment directed to the prevention of atelectasis should be administered before, during, and after anaesthesia. Adequate preoperative preparation of the patient is mandatory. Respiratory infections must be treated. Postural drainage and coughing exercises during the preceding 24 hours are desirable for those patients with sputum. The chest should be auscultated after tracheal intubation to ensure adequate aeration of both lungs, and adequate ventilation is required at all times during the anaesthetic period. Excess mucus should be frequently removed by suction. At the end of the anaesthetic coughing on the tracheal tube may loosen mucous plugs which may then be readily removed by suction.

During the postoperative period deep breathing exercises, frequent changes of position, and encouragement to cough will prevent atelectasis in most patients. Particular attention must be paid to obese and debilitated patients and to those with chronic lung disease. If atelectasis occurs,, coughing, deep breathing, and pounding on the affected side of the chest may be all that is necessary to release a mucous plug and effect a re-expansion of the lung. If atelectasis persists, bronchial suction through a tracheal tube or bronchoscope may be necessary. Atelectasis due to a foreign body in the bronchial tree will require bronchoscopy.

Pulmonary Oedema

Pulmonary oedema usually occurs suddenly in patients who have hypertension and cardiac disease, some of whom may have a history of cardiac failure. Pulmonary oedema may also be seen in normal patients who have been given excessive quantities of intravenous salt solutions. Ventilation becomes inadequate. There is increasing cyanosis, tachycardia, and a drop in blood pressure. Frothy blood-tinged fluid may be aspirated from the tracheal tube. Intravenous fluid intake must be carefully assessed in patients who have damaged hearts, to avoid the occurrence of pulmonary oedema.

Treatments consist of positive pressure breathing, rapid digitalization, and application of venous tourniquets or venesection.

Respiratory Arrest (Apnoea)

Cessation of breathing may be caused by depression or inhibition of the activity of the respiratory neurones in the central nervous system (respiratory centre) or paralysis of the respiratory muscles.

The neurones of the respiratory centre may be depressed by overdoses of narcotics, sedative drugs, or anaesthetic agents and by pathologically raised intracranial pressure. The rhythmic discharge of impulses by the respiratory neurones may be inhibited by reflexes arising from abdominal viscera, the trachea and bronchi, and by depression of the Hering-Breuer reflex and the reduction of P_{CO_2} during hyperventilation and assisted breathing. Paralysis of the muscles of respiration associated with anaesthesia may be due to disease processes, disturbances of electrolyte balance, or the action of muscle relaxants or high spinal anaesthesia.

The patient's history should be reviewed for evidence of muscle weakness (myasthenia gravis), carcinoma of the lung, hepatic or renal disease, or malnutrition. A clue to the cause of apnoea may be found in laboratory findings of low potassium or calcium. The anaesthetist should investigate the previous use of antibiotics (neomycin or streptomycin), large doses of narcotics, barbiturates, and hexamethonium compounds which, if given before or during anaesthesia, predispose to apnoea.

Apnoea caused by depression of the respiratory centres may require the use of opiate antagonists or respiratory stimulants. Inhibition of the centre by reflexes arising from the abdomen or respiratory tract is temporary and the treatment is to remove the stimulus. Inhibition of the respiratory centre by lowering of the P_{CO_2} due to hyperventilation will usually be reversed by decreasing the frequency and depth of respiration, thus allowing the P_{CO_2} to increase again to the threshold level for stimulation of the centre. Respiratory arrest due to intracranial pressure will only be reversed by treatment of the cause of the increased pressure.

Prolonged apnoea due to paralysis of the respiratory muscles usually occurs following the use of muscle relaxants, but may be caused or enhanced by hypokalaemia or the use of certain anti-biotics. Ether also has a synergistic action with the competitive blocking muscle relaxants.

Streptomycin, neomycin, and the polymyxin group of antibiotics have definite neuromuscular blocking properties, especially when given intraperitoneally or intravenously. Prolonged apnoea has also been reported following the use of muscle relaxants in cancer patients receiving AV-132.

The treatment of a persistent apnoea at the end of operation will depend on identification of the cause. In all events adequate ventilation must be maintained until the patient is able to breathe for himself. If a competitive blocking (non-depolarizing) muscle relaxant has been used throughout the operation, failure to reverse the block by the use of neostigmine (prostigmine) will in most cases be the result of poor peripheral vascular perfusion or acidosis. Gallamine is entirely excreted by the kidney, and will be retained by patients in renal failure.

Where a depolarizing relaxant has been used during operation, a dual block may be present (cf. chapter 5). Prolonged action of succinylcholine may be due to a genetic abnormality of plasma cholinesterase, or reduction of esterase levels in hepatic disease and malnutrition. Termination of the action of succinylcholine in such cases is determined by dilution and excretion, and ventilation must be maintained until this can occur.

When the suspicion exists that prolonged apnoea is due to the action of muscle relaxants, the nature of the block should be determined by the use of an electric stimulator on the ulnar nerve (cf. chapter 5).

CARDIOVASCULAR COMPLICATIONS

Any type of cardiovascular disturbance can occur in association with anaesthesia. Pre-existing hypertension or arteriosclerotic, rheumatic, or congenital heart disease or vascular disease may set the stage for untoward events when an anaesthetic is superimposed. Cardiovascular decompensation may be the result of pre-operative deficits of blood volume, electrolyte imbalance, anaemia, or previously administered drugs.

Hypotension and cardiac arrhythmias are commonly seen during anaesthesia. Hypertension occurs less commonly. Cardiac failure may occur in varying degrees, the most serious, of course, being cardiac arrest. The most common precipitating cause of cardiovascular complications is hypoxia.

Mechanisms controlling the circulation and the influence of anaesthesia upon these have been discussed in chapter 9.

Cardiac Arrhythmias

Cardiac arrhythmias occur frequently under anaesthesia; most are transient and do not seriously influence the function of the heart. Many may be detected only by the use of the electrocardiogram. More serious arrhythmias do occur, however, and require active treatment. Rational treatment will depend on identification of the underlying cause, whether this be unrecognized hypoxia, response to a reflex, or drug effect. As age is no longer a contraindication to surgery, many patients with cardiovascular disease and with reduced cardiac reserve may be presented for anaesthesia. In these patients disturbances of rhythm are more likely to occur and are more hazardous. The occurrence of these arrhythmias in response to anaesthesia has been discussed in chapter 9.

Air Embolism

Air embolism is particularly likely to occur in surgery with the patient in the sitting position, where a negative pressure develops in the veins of the head and neck as compared with the normal right atrial pressure, and air may be sucked into the venous system. The danger will be increased by a drop in venous pressure resulting from shock, haemorrhage, or hypotensive episodes. The air enters the vein during inspiration or may be forced in by external pressure. Air embolism may occur during surgery in the region of the veins in the head and neck, during pulmonary or intracardiac operations involving extracorporeal circulation, or during diagnostic procedures such as air insufflation studies.

Therapeutic procedures may also produce air embolism. It may occur for instance during vaginal insufflation with a powder blower, during establishment of pneumoperitoneum and artificial pneumothorax, or when air under pressure is used to speed transfusion. Angiography, trauma, abortions, and obstetrical procedures may also produce air embolism.

The air follows the venous circulation from the site of entry to the right ventricle, where the production of foam causes obstruction to the pulmonary outflow. The pulmonary flow requires approximately 50 per cent more time to pass through the capillaries of the lung than does blood alone, and there is also an incomplete emptying of the ventricle so that a residue of foamy blood remains after systole. Venous pressure rises and the right ventricle fails.

The introduction of air into the venous system may be indicated by an audible sucking sound as the air is drawn in. Air in the chambers of the heart produces a characteristic continuous murmur, described as a 'millwheel' murmur. In the patient who is breathing spontaneously respiration becomes irregular and gasping with the development of cyanosis. The pulse is thready, the blood pressure falls precipitously, and cardiac arrest may occur very quickly.

Treatment must be instituted immediately. Positive pressure should be applied to the airway using 100 per cent oxygen. The patient is turned head down in a steep Trendelenburg position with the right side uppermost. The anaesthetic is discontinued. If air is heard within the heart an attempt must be made to aspirate it. If the heart stops, cardiac massage must be instituted. The head-down position may prevent air emboli from entering the cerebral and coronary circulations.

Fat Embolism
Fat embolism may be associated with trauma to tissues in any part of the body, but is more common in association with fractures of the

long bones. This association with trauma to the long bones occurs because of the hollow fat-containing marrow cavity, and because the rigid support offered by the bone does not allow the veins to collapse. Fat passes into the opened veins as emboli which, after passing through the heart and pulmonary circulation, may reach the systemic circulation. Occlusion of the capillaries in the kidney, spleen, liver, and brain may follow. Cardiac arrest will occur when emboli enter the coronary arteries, or when acute cor pulmonale results from obstruction of the pulmonary circulation. Fat embolism may thus be a cause of unexpected death under anaesthesia.

Fat embolism may occur up to three or four days after trauma. In the awake patient apprehension is common, associated with rapid and laboured breathing, cyanosis, a rapid pulse, and temperature rising to 39° to 40° C. Signs of pulmonary oedema will be present, with basal rales and right-sided heart failure. There may be yellowish sputum. The patient may become unconscious or may show focal signs suggesting head injury.

Fat embolism is very difficult to diagnose. A chest X-ray shows diffuse cloudiness of the lungs, but is difficult to differentiate from other types of pulmonary oedema. A definite diagnosis may be made by laboratory studies of the urine stained with Sudan III, which in most cases will demonstrate the presence of fat. A dark field examination of serum for lipids may show droplets of fat.

Treatment is symptomatic. The pulmonary effects may be treated by pressure breathing with oxygen and other measures which are useful in the presence of pulmonary oedema and right-sided heart failure.

MALIGNANT HYPERTHERMIA

The occasional occurrence of a severe hyperpyrexial reaction during anaesthesia with potent agents has recently been recognized as a distinct and highly lethal syndrome with a hereditary basis, which is now called malignant hyperthermia. It has occurred in association with all the potent anaesthetic agents and at all ages. The cause appears to be metabolic defect in the muscle cell, the nature of which is not yet fully elucidated. Families in which this trait appears seem also to have a higher than normal incidence of other muscle disorders.

Two types of the malignant hyperthermia syndrome are recognized and these are described as the 'Rigid' and 'Non-rigid' types. The first type is characterized by generalized muscle rigidity which develops slowly under the influence of potent general anaesthetic agents in association with the developing hyperthermia, or which may typically be triggered by the administration of a depolarizing muscle relaxant such as succinylcholine, which produces prolonged rigidity and no relaxation in these patients. This rigidity is not influenced by competitive blocking relaxants such as tubocurarine.

No certain method currently exists for the detection of individuals affected by this trait. Where there is a family history of sudden death under anaesthesia, every member of that family should be considered to be at risk. Affected individuals may have a history of muscle cramps and may show unusually high levels of plasma creatine phosphokinase (CPK) after exertion, but normal CPK levels have been found in some survivors of Malignant Hyperthermia episodes.

Individuals in whom the trait is suspected may be anaesthetized with nitrous oxide and narcotic drugs, avoiding the use of muscle relaxants; or by regional anaesthetic techniques, preferably with procaine. The xylidide group of local anaesthetics is to be avoided, since these drugs may trigger an episode of malignant hyperthermia.

The body temperature in malignant hyperthermia reaches extreme levels, and has been recorded as high as 44.4° C (112° F) in some cases. These patients suffer hypoxia due to excessive metabolic demand for oxygen, extreme hypercarbia, and severe metabolic and respiratory acidosis. Muscle cells are destroyed, and early extreme hyperkalaemia is followed by total body hypokalaemia as potassium is excreted. The urine contains large amounts of myoglobin. Diffuse intravascular clotting may occur and bleeding follows due to consumption of clotting factors.

The occurrence of this syndrome may best be recognized by monitoring of the body temperature, and this is recommended as routine procedure during all but the briefest anaesthetics. Where rise in body temperature is not detected by such monitoring, the first signs of the syndrome are unexplained tachycardia and cyanosis, perhaps associated with developing rigidity.

Treatment must be prompt and vigorous. All anaesthetic agents must be immediately withdrawn, and the patient must be vigorously hyperventilated with high flows of oxygen through a tracheal tube. No reliance should be placed on soda-lime absorbers for the removal of carbon dioxide because their capacity will become quickly exhausted by the large quanties of CO_2 and the exothermic reaction of CO_2 absorption adds heat to the system. External cooling should be instituted by application of ice or a cooling blanket to the skin or immersion in ice water.

The immediate administration of procaine amide (Pronestyl®) 1000 mgm is recommended. This drug stabilizes the membrane of the sarcoplasmic reticulum of the muscle cell, and will promptly halt the process in the rigid type of malignant hyperthermia. Measurement of blood gases and electrolytes and appropriate regulation of acid/base balance and electrolyte concentrations are urgent and immediate requirements and, if the patient survives the episode, these will require careful assessment and regulation over several succeeding days. The principles of such management are discussed elsewhere in this manual.

TOXIC REACTIONS TO LOCAL ANAESTHESIA

Untoward reactions to local anaesthetic drugs may result from absolute overdose, hypersensitivity, or idiosyncrasy. Hypersensitivity may be defined as the usual type of reaction to a drug, but as a response to doses which would not usually prove to be toxic. Idiosyncrasy is an abnormal or unusual type of reaction to a drug.

Toxic reactions to local anaesthetic agents vary from tachycardia and minor nervous system irritation to convulsions and sudden respiratory and cardiac collapse. In the usual patient, systemic effects are associated with high blood levels, and are more pronounced after intravenous injections and topical applications to the mucous membranes of the respiratory tract. Absolute dosage of the drug is therefore important. The concentration of the drug is important too, since diffusion into the blood stream will be more rapid when higher concentrations are used.

The vascularity of the area of injection has importance in determining the rapidity of absorption into the blood stream. While the intravenous route is the most dangerous, absorption from the nasal, pharyngeal, tracheal, and bronchial mucosa produces high blood concentrations almost as rapidly because of the dense vascular system.

Before using a local anaesthetic drug, inquire specifically for a history of reaction to any previous local anaesthetic or a history of allergy to drugs and antitoxins. Most patients have had a local anaesthetic for dental procedures. If minor reactions have occurred, it is wise to prepare the patient by giving a barbiturate. Barbiturates will allay apprehension and the minor reactions associated with anaesthesia, as well as the sweating, tachycardia, and palpitation associated with too rapid absorption of adrenaline. Adrenaline is commonly used in association with local anaesthetics to slow the absorption and to prolong the action.

The smallest anaesthetic dose needed for an efficient block should be used. Using procaine as a standard, the maximum quantity to be used is 1 gm, i.e. 50 cc, of a 2 per cent solution, 100 cc of a 1 per cent solution, or 200 cc of a ½ per cent solution. As lidocaine is twice as potent as procaine, half the amount should be used. Smaller doses are given to very young, old, or debilitated patients.

If convulsions occur they must be immediately controlled with thiopentone intravenously, and artificial ventilation with oxygen must be initiated to combat cerebral anoxia.

Hypotension and a weak pulse may require the use of a vasopressor (e.g. phenylephrine or methoxamine). If there is a complete circulatory and respiratory collapse, cardiac massage and artificial ventilation with oxygen must be continued until an effective beat is restored.

True allergic responses are rare but may occur in patients who have a known hypersensitivity. Rarely, hypersensitivity may develop after a series of injections. However, allergic reactions will occur rapidly in already hypersensitive patients after a small dose, and therefore such patients should be given a test dose.

Gangrene may occur after injections of a local anaesthetic solution with adrenaline into the fingers or toes. No vasoconstrictor should be used in these areas, and after any injection these areas should be gently massaged.

CROSS-INFECTION AS A COMPLICATION
OF ANAESTHESIA

Considerable attention has been given to the role of anaesthetic equipment in spreading bacteria from one patient to another. During busy anaesthetic schedules patients appear in the theatres suffering from respiratory disease, sore throats, or infected mouths, and it is therefore wise to use special precautions with such patients. The anaesthetist should not administer anaesthetics if he himself is suffering from an acute respiratory disease, since he is liable to pass the infection along to the patient. Masks and caps should be worn and changed after every case.

Gas machines, especially the table tops, should be washed off with soap and water after every case, since they may be grossly contaminated by unsterile laryngoscopes, suction catheters, and endotracheal tubes. It is always wise to have a separate anaesthetic table for this equipment. Airways and endotracheal tubes should be placed in an unsterile container after use and resterilized. Fresh sterile towels should be placed on top of the gas machine and anaesthetic table before each case.

Preparation of the skin area for nerve block or spinal or epidural anaesthesia should be done as carefully as if one were preparing to make an incision. Needles should not enter the skin near an infected area showing pimples or pustules. Infection introduced into the spinal canal may cause a fatal meningitis. Similarly, the epidural space may become infected and create an epidural abscess.

Strict asepsis must be maintained in giving drugs intravenously. Multidose vials which may become contaminated by many aspirations are hazardous and should be avoided.

Sterilization of Anaesthetic Equipment
Anaesthetic equipment should be sterilized so that the danger of

cross infection will be minimal. Airways, tracheal tubes, face masks, and conductive rubber tubing deteriorate with autoclaving, and chemical methods of sterilization must be used. The method of choice is ethylene oxide, which is expensive and requires a special gas autoclave. It is also a slow process, but it does not damage any equipment that might be placed in it. Perhaps the best way of all would be to have a large gas autoclave that one could put the whole gas machine in.

Care of equipment after sterilization is just as important, and it is recommended that sterile plastic bags be used for storage. If ethylene oxide sterilization is not available the face masks may be thoroughly cleaned, rinsed, and hung up to dry unless the patient has been suffering from one of the more serious diseases such as tuberculosis. Special methods must be used for the tubercule bacillus and sporing bacteria. The usual methods used for sterilization are heat and chemicals. Airways, tracheal tubes, suction catheters, and other smaller items of equipment should be thoroughly cleaned and scrubbed with soap and water using bristled malleable brushes, then washed with sterile water and soaked for twelve hours in an antiseptic solution such as Zephirin®.

SORE THROAT

Sore throat is a common complaint during the postoperative period and may be due to several factors:

1 A throat pack soaked in water which remains rough and excoriates the mucous membrane of the throat.

2 Traumatic intubation The blade of the laryngoscope may cut the pharyngeal wall after too many attempts at intubation and traumatize the throat.

3 Prolonged coughing on tracheal tubes and airways.

4 Using too large a tracheal tube or overinflating the cuff.

5 Topical anaesthesia which may have an adverse effect.

6 Unsterile airways and tubes.

7 Pressure or traumatic introduction of stomach tubes.

8 Too vigorous pharyngeal suction during anaesthesia or in the postoperative period.

The above causes should be avoided where possible. Steam inhalations and throat gargles may be of some value in treatment. Antiallergic drugs may be indicated.

INTRA-ARTERIAL INJECTIONS

Intra-arterial injections of irritating solutions, including barbiturates (e.g. thiopentone) result in agonizing burning pain locally with blanching of the area supplied by that artery. The usual sites of such an accidental injection are in the antecubital fossa, on the dorsum of the hand, and at the wrist, due to abnormal ulnar or radial arteries.

The anaesthetist should feel for pulsation before using a 'vein' for injection. A test dose of 1 or 2 cc should always be used. If pain is elicited the injection should be stopped and procaine injected in and around the artery to relieve spasm. It may be necessary to do a stellate ganglion block. This treatment may have to be repeated.

Extravascular injections may cause neuritis or ulceration of the skin. Procaine 1 per cent or hyaluronidase injected around the area will relieve pain, dilute the irritant solution, and facilitate its removal from the issue.

EYE COMPLICATIONS

Eye complications are not as frequent now as they formerly were when chloroform and ether were administered by the open drop method. Ether is very irritating to the eye and may produce a severe burn or painful corneal ulcers.

Pressure from too large a mask over the eyes or from a headrest may cause severe pain and discomfort in the postoperative period as well as injury to the eye including blindness, and injury to the supraorbital nerves.

Pressure on the eye must be avoided. The eyelids should be closed and the eyes covered with a towel or rubber covering. Drops of protective solution should be instilled into the eye. Oily solutions should not be used since some anaesthetic vapours are absorbed by the oil. Antibiotics instilled locally will assist in healing abrasions and traumatic ulcers.

PERIPHERAL NERVE COMPLICATIONS

During anaesthesia, the anaesthetist must prevent injury to the peripheral nerves caused by the stretching and compression of nerves in the relaxed patient who is unable to complain of pain.

Stretching of the brachial plexus with resulting paralysis of the muscles of the arm may occur if the arm is abducted and externally rotated during a long operation, or if the arm is pulled above the head. The use of the Trendelenburg position combined with shoulder rests increases the likelihood of this injury by depressing the shoulder girdle.

Peripheral nerves may be injured by direct pressure during prolonged operations. Paralysis produced in this way is particularly likely to occur in the ulnar nerve as a result of pressure in the olecranon fossa by the edge of an operating table or mattress; to the common peroneal nerve by pressure of a lithotomy stirrup over the neck of the fibula; to the facial nerve by pressure of a head strap. Other possible nerve injuries and their causes are: median – injection of thiopentone or other irritating solution around the nerve; radial – arm falling off operating table, injection of drugs into the lateral side of the arm or into the antecubital fossa; saphenous – pressure; sciatic – intramuscular injections; pudendal – pressure; femoral – injury by retractors in gynaecological operations; obturator – obstetrical forceps; optic – pressure on eyeball, especially in prone position from headrests, pressure of ill-fitting masks; supraorbital – pressure of masks and tracheal tube connectors; abducens – spinal anaesthesia.

Spinal anaesthesia, local injections, and tourniquets can produce nerve injury. Cranial nerve lesions may be caused by slow dural leak which permits a descent of the medulla and pons and a resulting stretching of the cranial nerves. Tourniquets, if applied over a long period of time in relaxed patients, may injure nerves by compression. It is recommended that tourniquets be loosened every hour.

Trigeminal anaesthesia has been produced by breakdown products formed by the use of trichlorethylene in the presence of hot soda lime. Dichloracetylene formed in this way is very toxic to the central nervous system as a whole and may produce a general encephalopathy.

Nerve injuries should be prevented. Prolonged use of steep Trendelenburg position should be avoided. The arm should never be abducted at the shoulder beyond about 60° from the body, and supination should never be combined with such abduction. All areas where pressure may be applied to nerves should be adequately padded. Well-fitted face masks should be used and the eyes must be protected. The position of the patient on the table must be checked frequently. Injections near nerves, including nerve blocks, should be done with extreme caution.

The severity of nerve injury varies with the amount of stretching and compression that has been applied to the nerve and the duration of such trauma. Treatment may be necessary for many months and the condition may even require operative interference. Physiotherapy should be instituted immediately on making the diagnosis, to maintain the activity of muscles. This may require splinting, massage, galvanic current stimulation, and passive and active exercise.

ANAESTHETIC EXPLOSIONS

An anaesthetic explosion causing the death of a patient is a tragic and avoidable accident. Explosions are infrequent and one may say that they are relatively insignificant as compared with other hazards. New non-explosive anaesthetic agents like halothane and methoxyflurane have helped to reduce the hazard.

The obvious sources of ignition are alcohol lamps, cigarettes, matches, leaky anaesthetic machines, defective wiring, and static electricity.

Electric wiring must conform to the National Electric Code and the National Board of Fire Underwriters and Canadian Standards Association codes. Explosion-proof switches, spark-proof enclosed motors, and grounded conduits must always be used in operating rooms. Kinkless and rubber-coated cords are desirable. Antistatic materials must be used for floors and equipment in anaesthetic rooms and operating theatres. Conductive footwear must be worn by all personnel. The use of woollen and nylon blankets must be prohibited. No cautery may be used in conjunction with flammable or explosive anaesthetic agents. The ether bottle and the tank of cyclopropane should be removed from the anaesthetic machine when a source of ignition such as an electrocautery is to be present during an operation.

Static sparks are the greatest hidden source of ignition, and considerable research has been carried out over the years directed to eliminating this hazard. To avoid ignition from this source all anaesthetic equipment or attachments that have contact with the patient must be of conductive material. Furniture and operating tables must make contact with conductive floors by metal or conductive rubber casters. The humidity of the operating room should be above 50 per cent to reduce the danger of static sparks.

Rooms should be well ventilated to prevent the accumulation of explosive gases. The closed system of administering anaesthetic agents lessens the danger of static sparks from outside the area but this does not mean that protection will be complete. It is generally agreed that the area around the patient's head and the anaesthetic apparatus presents the greatest source of danger owing to a heavier concentration of the explosive agent there. Making and breaking metal-to-metal connections near the head should be carried out only after equalizing static charges, and the flow of anaesthetic gases should be discontinued during this period.

COMPLICATIONS OF SPINAL ANAESTHESIA

The common complications met during spinal anaesthesia are hypotension and respiratory paralysis, which have been discussed earlier in this chapter. Restlessness due to cerebral hypoxia associated with hypotension or depression of ventilation should not be confused with apprehension. Nausea and vomiting may also be a response to cerebral hypoxia associated with hypotension and anoxia, or it may result from vagal reflexes from the viscera, which are not blocked by spinal anaesthesia. These complications should all be avoided by proper attention to ventilation, and the control of hypotension by the judicious use of small intravenous doses of vasopressor drugs. Later complications of spinal anaesthesia are headaches, arachnoiditis, meningitis, radiculitis, neuritis, paraplegia, cauda equina syndrome, and the neurogenic bladder. With the exception of headaches, these complications are rare.

Persistent headache commonly seen after spinal anaesthesia appears to be due to the leakage of spinal fluid from the dura at the site of puncture. This leak creates a low fluid pressure in the spinal theca which may drag on the sensitive parts of the brain and its attachments. The greater incidence of headache when larger needles are used supports this theory. The incidence of postspinal headache may be greatly reduced by using fine-gauge spinal needles (e.g. 26 gauge). Some headaches are undoubtedly due to other causes, and headache associated with meningismus may occur due to irritation of the meninges by bacterial or chemical contaminants from needles and syringes cleaned with tap water or with cleaning solutions. Such irritation may be avoided by thorough cleansing of all equipment with distilled water before sterilization.

The usual treatment of postspinal headache consists of hydration by the administration of appropriate intravenous fluids, the use of mild analgesics such as aspirin, and keeping the patient flat on his back without a pillow for 12 to 24 hours or more. In severe cases the injection of 40 to 50 cc of physiological saline solution into the subarachnoid space or the epidural space may provide relief.

Paraplegia occurring after spinal anaesthesia is thought to be due to the injection of solutions contaminated with chemical sterilizing agents. Ampoules of drugs to be used in spinal anaesthesia should always be sterilized by autoclaving.

Complications of epidural anaesthesia are fewer and consist mainly of hypotension, painful back, and occasional headache.

CONVULSIONS COMPLICATING ANAESTHESIA

Convulsions occurring as a manifestation of the toxicity of local anaesthetics have already been discussed. Convulsions may also occur in association with general anaesthesia, and have been more common in children receiving ethyl or vinyl ether than in adults. The occurrence of such convulsions is almost universally associated with dehydration, acidosis, and a high fever in an infant or child. The incidence should be very rare indeed if patients are properly prepared for operation. Cerebral anoxia and accumulation of carbon dioxide may also have some significance in causing these convulsions.

When such a convulsion occurs, the anaesthetic should be discontinued and the patient should be well ventilated with oxygen and given a muscle relaxant, if necessary, to control the convulsion. Body temperature should be reduced. It has been suggested that the intravenous administration of calcium salts may be effective.

REFERENCES

ADAMS, AILEEN. Information and Misinformation from the E.K.G. during Anaesthesia. *19*: 585 (1964)

ADRIANI, JOHN. Appraisal of Current Concepts in Anesthesiology, chapter 28. St. Louis: Mosby (1961)

ADRIANI, J.; CAMPBELL, D.; & YARBERRY, O.H. Influence of Absorption on Systemic Toxicity of Local Anesthetic Agents. Anesthesia and Analgesia. *38*: 370 (1959)

ARGENT, D.E.; DINNICK, O.P.; & HOBBIGER, F. Prolonged Apnoea after Suxamethonium in Man. British Journal of Anaesthesia. *27*: 24 (1955)

BANNISTER, W.K. & SALTILARO, A.J. Vomiting and Aspiration during Anesthesia. Anesthesiology. *23*: 251 (1962)

BOURNE, J.G. Anesthesia and the Vomiting Hazard. Anaesthesia. *17*: 379 (1962)

BOYAN, C.P. & HOWLAND, W.S. Cardiac Arrest and Temperature of Bank Blood, Journal of the American Medical Association. *183*: 58 (1963)

BRACHAN, S. Explosion Risk in a Non-flammable System. Anaesthesia. *18*: 439 (1963)

BRENNAN, H.J. Dual Action of Suxamethonium. British Journal of Anaesthesia. *28*: 59 (1956)

BRITT, B.A. & GORDON, R.A. Peripheral Nerve Injuries Associated with Anaesthesia. Canadian Anaesthetists' Society Journal. *11*: 514 (1964)

CONVERSE, J.G. & SMOTRILLA, M.M. Anesthesia and the Asthmatic. Anesthesia and Analgesia. *40*: 336 (1961)

CONWAY, C.M.; MILLER, J.S.; & SUGDEN, F.L.H. Sore Throat after Anaesthesia. British Journal of Anaesthesia. *32*: 319 (1960)

DALE, W.A. Cardiac Arrest: Review and Report of 12 Cases. Annals of Surgery. *135*: 376 (1952)

DAVENPORT, H.T. & KEENLEYSIDE, H.B. Interstitial Emphysema and Pneumothorax Associated with the Use of a Modified Non-rebreathing Valve. Canadian Anaesthetists' Society Journal. *4*: 126 (1957)

DORNETTE, W.H.L. & HUGHES, B.H. Care of the Teeth during Anesthesia. Anesthesia and Analgesia. *38*: 206 (1959)

DRIPPS, R.D.; ECKENHOFF, J.E.; & VANDAM, L.D. Introduction to Anesthesia. 2nd ed., chapters 14, 18, 35, London, Philadelphia: Saunders (1961)

EDWARDS, G.; MORTON, H.J.V.; PASK, E.A.; & WYLIE, W.D. Deaths associated with Anaesthesia. Anaesthesia. *11*: 194 (1956)

EMERY, E.R.J. Neuromuscular Blocking Properties of Antibiotics as a Cause of Postoperative Apnoea. Anaesthesia. *18*: 57 (1963)

ENDOVE, H.S.; LEVIN, M.J.; & RANT-SEJDINAJ, IRENE. Neurological Complications of Spinal Anaesthesia. Canadian Anaesthetists' Society Journal. *8*: 405 (1961)

FELDMAN, S.A. & LEVI, J.A. Prolonged Paresis following Gallamine. British Journal of Anaesthesia. *35*: 804 (1963)

GARDNER, A.M.N. Aspiration of Food and Vomitus. Quarterly Journal of Medicine. *27*: 227 (1958)

GILBERT, R.G.B. Neurological Complications of Spinal Anaesthesia. Canadian Anaesthetists' Society Journal. *2*: 116 (1955)

GORDON, R.A.; BRITT, B.A.; & KALOW, W. (Eds). International Symposium on Malignant Hyperthermia, Springfield, Charles C. Thomas, 1973.

GRENNELL, H.A. & VANDEWATER, S.L. The Supine Hypotensive Syndrome during Conduction Anaesthesia for the Near-Term Gravid Patient: Case Reports. Canadian Anaesthetists' Society Journal, *8*: 4 (1961)

HARTSELL, C.J. & STEPHEN, C.R. Incidence of Sore Throat following Endotracheal Intubation. Canadian Anaesthetists' Society Journal. *11*: 307 (1964)

HAUGEN, F.P. Symposium: Post-anesthetic Complication. Anesthesiology. *22*: 657 (1961)

KATZ, R.L.; WOLF, C.E.; & PAPPER, E.M. The Nondepolarizing Neuromuscular Blocking Action of Succinylcholine in Man. Anesthesiology. *24*: 784 (1963)

KEATING, V. Anesthetic Accidents. 2nd ed., chapters 1, 11, Chicago: Year Book Publishers (1961)

KYLE, W.D. Acute Pulmonary Collapse: A Case Report. Canadian Anaesthetists' Society Journal. *10*: 550 (1963)

LEWIS, R.N. & SWERDLOW, M. Hazards of Endotracheal Anaesthesia. British Journal of Anaesthesia. *36*: 504 (1964)

MARSHALL, B.M. & GORDON, R.A. Vomiting, Regurgitation, and Aspiration in Anaesthesia: I. Canadian Anaesthetists' Society Journal. *5*: 274 (1958)

—— Vomiting, Regurgitation, and Aspiration in Anaesthesia: II. Canadian Anaesthetists' Society Journal. *5*: 438 (1958)

MARTIN, J.T. & PATRICK, R.T. Pneumothorax: Its Significance to the Anesthesiologist. Anesthesia and Analgesia. *39*: 420 (1960)

MARTIN, S.J. Consideration of the Etiology and Treatment of Sudden Cardiac Collapse. Anesthesia and Analgesia. *39*: 23 (1960)

MCKERSIE, W.G. Spinal Anaesthesia: A Re-evaluation. Canadian Anaesthetists' Society Journal. *3*: 117 (1956)

MERRILL, R.B. & HINGSON, R.A. Study of Incidence of Maternal Mortality from Aspiration Vomitus during Anaesthesia Occurring in Major Obstetric Hospital in United States. Anesthesia and Analgesia. *30*: 121 (1951)

MINUCK, MAX. The Chemotherapy of Cardiac Arrest. Canadian Medical Association Journal. *92*: 16 (1965)

MUCKLOW, R.G. & LARARD, D. The Effects of the Inhalation of Vomitus on the Lungs: Clinical Considerations. British Journal of Anaesthesia. *35*: 153 (1965)

RUSTON, F.G. & POLITI, V.L. Femoral Nerve Injury from Abdominal Retractors. Canadian Anaesthetists' Society Journal. *5*: 428 (1958)

SHUMACKER, H.B. & HAMPTON, L.S. Sudden Death Occurring Immediately after Operation in Patients with Cardiac Disease, with Particular Reference to the Role of Aspiration through the Endotracheal Tube and Extubation. Journal of Thoracic Surgery. *21*: 48 (1951)

STARK, D.C.; GREEN, C.A.; & PASK, E.A. Anaesthetic Machines and Cross Infection. Anaesthesia. *17*: 12 (1962)

STEPHEN, C.R.; MARTIN, R.; & NOWILL, W.K. How Safe is Spinal Anaesthesia in Present-Day Practice? North Carolina Medical Journal. *15*: 33 (1954)

STRATFORD, B.D.; CLARK, R.R.; & DIXSON, SHIRLEY. Disinfection of Anaesthetic Apparatus. British Journal of Anaesthesia. *36*: 471 (1964)

TAYLOR, G.J. Apnoea Due to Apparent Potassium Imbalance. Anaesthesia. *18*: 9 (1963)

VANDAM, L.D. & DRIPPS, R.D. Long-Term Follow-Up of Patients Who Received 10,098 Spinal Anaesthetics. Journal of the American Medical Association. *172*: 1483 (1960)

WATER, C.W. Anesthetic Explosions: A Continuing Threat. Anesthesiology. *25*: 505 (1964)

WOOD-SMITH, F.G. & STEWART, H.C. Drugs in Anaesthetic Practice. London: Butterworth (1962)

E.A. GAIN

13
Postoperative problems and care

Many problems arise in the early postoperative period; not all are the result of the anaesthetic, but many of them are usually cared for by the anaesthetist because they often occur while the patient is in the post-anaesthetic recovery room and still under the anaesthetist's supervision.

RESPIRATORY PROBLEMS

Respiratory problems are frequently encountered but are perhaps least often recognized.

Inadequate ventilation may result from central depression caused by excessive doses of central respiratory depressants such as opiates, barbiturates, and inhalation anaesthetic agents. The other common cause is residual muscle weakness as a result of muscle relaxants. Inadequate ventilation can only be determined by measuring the patient's tidal exchange, or, when possible, the arterial carbon dioxide tension. A high index of suspicion may be obtained by observing the nature of the patient's breathing. Colour is a poor indicator as cyanosis is a very late and unreliable sign of inadequate ventilation. Delayed recovery of consciousness should make the physician suspect inadequate ventilation with carbon dioxide accumulation unless another cause is proved. Depression of respiration due to opiates can be effectively counteracted by the use of appropriate antagonists, as can muscle weakness from residual muscle relaxant effect. When inadequate ventilation is the result of an overdose of barbiturate or an inhalation anaesthetic agent the only effective treatment is to assist the patient's ventilation by some artificial means, either manually with a mask and bag, or with one of the many machines available for the administration of intermittent positive pressure respiration, until these agents have been eliminated from the body.

Atelectasis is encountered much less often than in the past because of better preoperative preparation and better postoperative care. The usual obstructive atelectasis rarely has any relation to the anaesthetic agent or method, but is the result of excessive bronchial secretions which, because of pain from the operative site or the patient's inability or refusal to cough, produce obstruction in the bronchi with absorption of gases distal to the obstructing secretions. Atelectasis involving varying amounts of lung may result. As would be expected, atelectasis occurs more often after thoracic and upper abdominal surgery. It is seen more often in patients with chronic pulmonary disease such as bronchitis, emphysema, asthama, and in heavy smokers. Preventive measures should be instituted preoperatively in all patients who are likely to develop this complication. Preoperative postural drainage, aerosol bronchodilators and antibiotics, and the discontinuance of smoking preoperatively will markedly reduce the incidence of atelectasis. Preventive measures such as early ambulation, deep breathing and coughing – the so-called stir-up regimen – must be instituted early in the postoperative period.

Another likely cause of postoperative atelectasis is the indiscriminate postoperative use of narcotic analgesics. The normal individual takes frequent deep breaths or sighs to overcome the decreasing compliance which accompanies fixed volume ventilation. Patients under anaesthesia or heavy narcotic sedation fail to take deep breaths or to change the volume of their ventilation and therefore suffer a decrease in compliance from collapse of the peripheral areas of the lung caused by absorption of the soluble anaesthetic gases from these distal alveoli. It is therefore essential that patients who are receiving frequent doses of postoperative analgesics should be encouraged to take deep breaths at regular short intervals to prevent this form of atelectasis. Obstructive atelectasis usually manifests itself 24 to 72 hours postoperatively and the first indication may be a rise in pulse rate with a spiking temperature. Such findings on the patient's chart should make the physician suspect atelectasis as the most likely cause. The other classical signs such as tachypnoea, apprehension, tracheal shift, and absent breath sounds will depend for their appearance on the amount of atelectatic lung present. These signs may be absent altogether. Treatment of atelectasis consists of making the patient cough to clear obstructing secretion from the tracheobronchial tree. As a rule this is all that is required, but it may be necessary in some cases to stimulate the cough reflex by direct irritation of the tracheobronchial tree. In severely debilitated, comatose, or paralysed patients who are physically unable to clear their tracheobronchial tree, bronchoscopy with suction may have to be resorted to. It is most important that atelectasis be prevented, and if it should occur it must be quickly and vigorously treated as most instances of postoperative pneumonia occur secondary to atelectasis.

Aspiration pneumonitis is a complication that usually occurs during or at the immediate termination of anaesthesia. It has been considered in more detail in chapter 12. It may however occur at any time during the postoperative period, and these late cases are more likely to be seen in the elderly and debilitated patient. If such a patient has vomited in the postoperative period and is found to be dyspnoeic and possibly cyanotic, exhibiting tachycardia and restlessness, then the chest must be examined; if rales and rhonchi are heard a chest X-ray should be obtained and therapy commenced at once. Therapy consists of large doses of steroids. The use of antihistamines, aerosol bronchodilators, and antibiotics may be helpful. This condition carries a very high mortality rate if neglected.

Pneumothorax may result from excessive airway pressure applied by the anaesthetist either intentionally or unintentionally because of faulty equipment. Excess pressure causes alveolar rupture and the free gas tracks along the pulmonary vessels producing a mediastinal emphysema. This emphysema in turn may rupture through the mediastinal pleura thereby producing a pneumothorax. In rare instances reasonable airway pressure may cause rupture of congenital or emphysematous bullae directly into the pleural space. Although pneumothorax usually occurs during the anasthetic it is often unrecognized until the immediate postoperative period. The treatment required will vary with the cause and degree of respiratory and circulatory embarrassment which results. It is discussed more fully in chapter 12.

CIRCULATORY PROBLEMS

Circulatory problems are numerous, but most of them occur in the immediate postoperative period, again while the patient is still under the anaesthetist's care.

Hypotension A low systolic blood pressure is the most frequent problem and is often due to inadequate blood replacement during the operation. This produces hypovolaemia, manifested not only by low systolic blood pressure, but by tachycardia, small pulse pressure, pallor, and often the classical cold moist skin. Haemorrhage may often be concealed, as in thoracic and abdominal surgery, and it is frequently not appreciated that large amounts of blood can be lost into the tissues of the thigh and back from surgery in these areas. The treatment is blood replacement. If blood is not immediately available volume expanders may be used until blood can be obtained.

Another form of hypotension is that seen following pelvic and perineal surgery. The onset is usually about the time the patient commences to manifest discomfort from the operation; the systolic pressure is low, the pulse pressure very low, and the pulse is very slow. Usually the patient is pale, but the skin is warm and dry and the patient is not restless or apprehensive as is often the case with hypovolaemic shock. This hypotension with bradycardia is believed to result from irritation of the pelvic splanchnic nerves resulting in a vagal efferent reflex. Vagal stimulation causes bradycardia, a decrease in the force of cardiac contraction, and vasodilatation. This condition may be corrected by blocking the excess vagal activity with intravenous atropine or by increasing sympathetic activity with a vasopressor drug with inotropic and chronotropic properties.

Hypotension is often encountered in the postoperative period in those patients who have received spinal or epidural anaesthesia. In this instance, sympathetic block with a loss of peripheral resistance has produced a condition closely resembling the hypotension following pelvic surgery, but the pulse rate with sympathetic block is usually normal or a slow-normal. An increase in peripheral resistance is required to correct this hypotension, and is obtained by the use of vasopressor agents. If a patient who has received spinal or epidural anaesthesia has a tachycardia with hypotension, then one must suspect that hypovolaemia is present also and the patient will require blood replacement.

Myocardial failure With the increasing age of the population more patients with degenerative cardiovascular disease are being presented for surgery. Consequently postoperative cardiac failure is becoming a more frequent problem. During well-administered anaesthesia few such problems arise because the cardiac patient under anaesthesia is often in a better state than he will be in the postoperative period. During anaesthesia there is little if any muscle activity, the oxygen requirements are below basal levels, and the heart has less work to perform. On recovery from anaesthesia the pain from the surgery causes an increase in muscle activity and therefore in the oxygen requirements. This places an added load on the heart, and myocardial ischaemia and failure not infrequently occur in the cardiac patient. The classical signs are usually present. There is peripheral cyanosis and not pallor, and venous jugular pressure is elevated and not decreased as with hypovolaemic hypotension. It is obvious therefore that fluids and blood must not be given; instead these patients require oxygen and digitalization. Fluid overload can easily occur during the operation if blood replacement has been too vigorous. Because of the frequent use of positive pressure ventilation during anaesthesia, fluid overload and heart failure may not be recognized unless venous pressures are monitored. This measurement is unlikely to be carried out under usual circumstances, thus only when the surgery and positive pressure ventilation terminate will the patient begin to show the signs of pulmonary oedema. Limb tourniquets or phlebotomy, digitalization, and possibly resumption of positive pressure ventilation will be required to control the oedema. It may be necessary in some severe cardiac patients to maintain artificial ventilation with an automatic ventilator for hours or even days to reduce the work load of the heart. The oxygen demand of the muscles of respiration can increase from the normal basal level of 1 to 2 per cent of the total oxygen requirement of the body to as high as 50 per cent in postoperative thoracic surgery patients. This represents a tremendous increase in the work load of the heart. If this load is not removed by artificial means many weakened or diseased hearts will fail.

In all instances of postoperative myocardial failure and cardiac arrhythmias, coronary insufficiency or occlusion should be suspected and an electrocardiogram obtained as myocardial ischaemia and hypoxia are a likely cause. This ischaemia or hypoxia may be due either to inadequate coronary flow or to pulmonary causes, and steps should be taken to increase coronary flow or raise the oxygen tension of the blood, or both, depending on whether the aetiology is coronary insufficiency or inadequate pulmonary ventilation.

GASTROINTESTINAL PROBLEMS

Gastrointestinal complications are not frequent during the immediate postoperative period when the patient is under the anaesthetist's care; they usually develop a few hours later.

Vomiting Nausea and vomiting have until recent times been considered a normal accompaniment of all anaesthetics, and anaesthesia is still believed by many to be the cause of most postoperative vomiting. This was undoubtedly true in the days of deep anaesthesia which was accompanied by respiratory and metabolic acidosis, ketosis, dehydration, and electrolyte disturbances. With the advent of muscle relaxants, light levels of anaesthesia, and close attention to ventilation, blood, fluid and electrolyte replacement, anaesthesia is today rarely responsible for any significant postoperative vomiting. The most frequent cause is surgical, either the direct result of the surgery or more often from the use of narcotic analgesic drugs given to relieve postoperative pain. If anaesthesia is properly conducted, and gastric and intestinal distension prevented by the use of suction, then the usual offender is the narcotic analgesic drug being used. Often the nausea and vomiting associated with the usual dose of morphine or meperidine can be eliminated by using one of the newer phenothiazine anti-emetics. Anti-emetic drugs should rarely be required, but when they are, the drugs of the penothiazine group are the most effective. When using anti-emetics of this type great care must be exercised, since many of these drugs potentiate the action of all sedatives and analgesics and in combination may cause severe respiratory and circulatory depression.

Gastric distension may be the result of over-enthusiastic efforts by the anaesthetist in carrying out artificial ventilation, with the result that excessive amounts of anaesthetic gases are forced into the stomach. Usually this is not of serious significance in the average adult patient, but it can be very serious in the infant. Respiratory and circulatory embarrassment may occur and these can be quickly and effectively relieved by the insertion of a stomach tube.

Acute gastric dilatation consists of a sudden distention of the stomach with gastric secretions, resulting in the sudden appearance of circulatory collapse. This may occur at any time in the postoperative period, usually after the patient has been returned to the care of the surgeon. Patients who have suffered circulatory collapse as a result of acute gastric dilatation may vomit enormous amounts of black-brown acidic gastric fluid and run the hazard of aspiration and the development of aspiration pneumonitis. Treatment requires the immediate recognition of this complication and the institution of continuous gastric suction and adequate fluid and electrolyte replacement.

HEPATIC PROBLEMS

Postoperative impairment of hepatic function may be due to any one or to a combination of several causes. These causes include surgical manipulation of the liver or its blood supply, shock or hypotension and the hepatotoxic action or interaction of drugs, including antibiotics and, perhaps, some anaesthetic agents. The possibility of coincidental infectious hepatitis or an exacerbation of chronic hepatitis must not be overlooked. The controversial problem of hepatitis associated with halothane anaesthesia is discussed in chapter 4.

RENAL PROBLEMS

Oliguria often follows anaesthesia and may result from excessive depth of anaesthesia, inadequate hydration, disordered electrolyte concentrations, prolonged renal ischaemia from shock.

High output renal failure may occur as a result of toxic effects of some drugs. Such renal failure has been documented following methoxyflurane anaesthesia, and is probably caused by free fluoride ion or other substances produced during the biodegradation of methoxyflurane (chapter 4).

Treatment of postoperative renal problems will depend on a correct diagnosis.

OTHER POSTOPERATIVE PROBLEMS

Hypothermia Inadvertent hypothermia is more frequently encountered today because of air-conditioned operating suites, prolonged surgery with abdominal and thoracic cavities open, and the use of large amounts of refrigerated blood. Hypothermia in the postoperative period leads to vasoconstriction and shivering, with the result that oxygen demands are increased and metabolic acidosis may result. In most adults hypothermia is not severe and the body temperature rapidly returns to normal. Such is not the case with the newborn and the very young infant. These patients can become hypothermic very rapidly, and the consequences are much more serious than in the adult. Small children have great difficulty in re-establishing normal body temperature, and when they are hypothermic their respiration is often inadequate. It has also been reported that hypothermia in the infant results in feeding difficulties in the postoperative period. Therefore steps must be taken during anaesthesia to prevent the development of this complication by providing suitable environmental temperature, avoiding prolonged surgery in the infant when possible, and by using warming mattresses under the patient and blood warmers when large amounts of refrigerated blood are required.

Delayed recovery of consciousness There are many causes for delay in recovery following anaesthesia, and many of them are the result of the surgery, particularly when neurosurgery is involved. Those causes associated with the anaesthesia are usually the result of anaesthetic overdose. If it is desirable to hasten recovery, then artificial means of increasing ventilation will be necessary to increase the elimination of inhalation anaesthetic agents. If the anaesthetic agent was a non-volatile one such as a barbiturate or narcotic, no usual methods will hasten the elimination. In all such cases of anaesthetic overdose, be it with inhalation or intravenous agents or muscle relaxants, the first step should be to determine the adequacy of ventilation, for this may be the primary cause in many instances of delayed recovery. Inadequate ventilation can rapidly produce carbon dioxide narcosis and/or hypoxia, and consciousness will not return until blood gases are restored to near normal levels by the application of artificial or associated methods of ventilation.

If severe cerebral ischaemia has occurred during operation, either from severe prolonged hypotension or from an actual cardiac standstill, cerebral hypoxia with resulting cerebral oedema may have occurred and may be the cause of the delayed return of consciousness. If recovery is prolonged or if signs of central nervous system irritability or hyperthermia occur, then steps must be instituted to treat the cerebral oedema. Osmotic diuretics and hypothermia may be employed to treat the cerebral oedema and the hyperthermia, and also to reduce the oxygen requirements of the brain. Cerebral acidosis and reduced cerebral oxygen tension may be improved by hyperventilation, which will increase the arterial oxygen tension and produce a compensatory respiratory alkalosis.

Shivering A frequent but usually benign complication and may be seen after all types of general anaesthesia. It may or may not be associated with a reduced temperature. It may be hazardous in some patients because of the increased oxygen requirements associated with it. It is usually readily controlled by the careful administration of intravenous opiates or sympatholytic sedatives.

Restlessness Often reaching the stage of confusion, excitement, and violence, restlessness requires sedation in most instances with drugs such as diazepam. When pain is the cause opiates are preferred. Hypoxia from inadequate ventilation must always be ruled out before treating restlessness with respiratory depressants.

Pain This is the most usual postoperative problem and should be treated with small intravenous doses of narcotic analgesics. The intravenous route is preferable as the dose can be more readily titrated to the patient's needs and any deleterious effects (such as respiratory depression) can be seen immediately. If narcotics are given by the intramuscular route, then small doses must be used and the patient observed for 45 minutes as absorption is slow. The action of narcotics is markedly potentiated by anaesthetic drugs and particularly the barbiturates. Large doses of narcotics may result in a patient becoming re-anaesthetized and even apnoeic with disastrous results should this occur back on the ward after the patient has left the recovery room.

S.L. VANDEWATER

14
Obstetrical anaesthesia
and resuscitation of the newborn

On January 19, 1847, James Young Simpson of Edinburgh administered ether for the first time to a woman in labour who required a version and breech extraction. Simpson at that time stated, 'I believe that as a counteraction to the morbific influence of pain, the state of artificial anaesthesia does not imply a saving of human suffering, but also a saving of human life.'

The problems that face us today are little different from those that faced Simpson over one hundred years ago. The question still raised is whether we protect or jeopardize the lives of mothers and infants by the administration of obstetric analgesia and anaesthesia. Investigations to date have failed to yield conclusive answers. During the past 25 years there has been a marked reduction in maternal and foetal morbidity and mortality due to vastly improved prenatal and obstetrical care, the availability of blood, the development of antibiotics, and a better understanding of toxaemias. The effects and complications of analgesia and anaesthesia, at one time a small factor in the complications of obstetrics, although still small, have increased in relative importance as the incidence and severity of haemorrhage, toxaemia, and infection have been reduced.

THE PLACENTA AS A BARRIER TO ANALGESICS
AND ANAESTHETICS

The placenta (which means a 'flat cake') in all mammals is the organ by which the blood streams of mother and foetus are brought into close association to facilitate exchange of nutrients and waste products. The two circulations are separated by three layers of foetal tissue which constitute a thin, semi-permeable membrane of considerable area, easily affected by the factors of osmosis, hydrostatic pressure, and diffusion gradients.

The role of the placenta has been likened to a foetal lung, as oxygen and carbon dioxide are transferred by rapid diffusion. Investigations in both animals and humans have shown that all drugs used for sedation and general anaesthesia, excepting some curariform drugs, cross the placental barrier by diffusion, the speed depending on molecular size, lipid solubility, electrical charge, and concentration gradient. Regardless of the route of administration – orally, by injection, or by inhalation – all narcotics, tranquillizers, barbiturates, and volatile and gaseous anaesthetics rapidly reach a concentration in the foetal blood paralleling and sometimes equaling that in the maternal blood.

OBSTETRICAL ANALGESIA AND ANAESTHESIA

During the past thirty years the medical press has carried numerous enthusiastic reports on the merits of various analgesics and hypnotics, and their apparent lack of foetal effects. A continuous and at times heated discussion has gone on between the proponents of general anaesthesia and those of conduction anaesthesia. Every drug with any conceivable application to obstetrical analgesia and anaesthesia has been described. The many different methods and agents recommended attest to the fact that none is ideal. Many drugs and methods of anaesthesia give good pain relief to the mother, but may depress the baby, whereas others do no harm to the infant, barring complications, but are unreliable (e.g. pudendal nerve block) or give inadequate pain relief, or require much technical skill (e.g. lumbar or sacral peridural block).

Analgesia

At present the drugs used for pain relief during labour are the synthetic morphine-like analgesics, meperidine (Demerol) 50–100 mg or alphaprodine (Nisentil) 20–40 mg, given either parenterally alone, or combined with hyoscine (0.4 mg) or a phenothiazine derivative such as promethazine (Phenergan) 25–50 mg. This is not to say that other narcotics (e.g. morphine or pantopon) cannot be used, but it must be remembered that though there may be slight differences as to time of onset and duration of action, and possibly differences in incidence of nausea and vomiting, they all produce about the same degree of respiratory depression if given in equi-analgesic doses. This depressant action is transferred to the foetus. Ideally narcotics should not be given within two hours of expected delivery time. If the mother is obviously depressed from narcotics just prior to delivery because of repeated use of these drugs, or a recent administration, then it would appear wise to inject a 'narcotic antagonist' intravenously, i.e., a drug which will reverse the respiratory depression, such as N-allylnormorphine (Nalline) 1–5 mg or levorphanol (Lorfan) 0.5–1.0 mg.

The hyoscine in the above-mentioned combination is used for its known amnesic action through cortical depression, not for its antisialogue effect (drying of secretions). Promethazine, primarily a potent antihistaminic drug, produces drowsiness, and is useful in combination with meperidine (Demerol) which does not have the euphoric action of morphine. In addition, promethazine has a moderate anti-emetic action, which is of some importance in relation to obstetrical anaesthesia. In prolonged labour, oral barbiturates will help to promote sleep.

The use of self-administered trichlorethylene (Trilene) with air has not been popular in this country, and prolonged administration may cause undue maternal and foetal depression. More recently, with the availability of skilled specialist anaesthetic services, continuous lumbar epidural analgesia (block at T 10–12 level) is receiving greater attention. This block can be reinforced intermittently for hours or even days and will provide anaesthesia for delivery. However, it is not to be undertaken except by those experienced and trained in its use, as severe complications can occur.

Analgesia is more commonly used in the primigravida. Finally, it must be remembered that the depressant effect may be potentiated by the subsequent administration of general anaesthetics, even in minimal concentrations.

Anaesthesia

The choice of anaesthetic agent and technique is to a large extent dictated by local obstetrical practice and availability of physician anaesthetic services. If a physician is unavailable to administer an anaesthetic, then anaesthesia should be limited to infiltration of the perineum or bilateral pudendal block with 1–2 per cent procaine or lignocaine (Xylocaine) not exceeding a total dose of 400 mg. The practice of the attending physician carrying out a spinal or epidural block and then delivering the patient is not recommended as safe. Having a nurse pour ether or chloroform on a mask, or use an anaesthetic machine, is condemned as hazardous and illegal.

A physician anaesthetist should choose a method and drug with which he is familiar and in keeping with the amount of sedation that is used and the type of delivery contemplated.

General anaesthesia No anaesthesia, local, conduction, or general, should be undertaken unless the means of administering oxygen under pressure is at hand, and the equipment understood. Open-drop ether given intermittently with uterine contraction has been successfully employed for many years, but modern anaesthetic equipment is now usually at hand in delivery rooms. For short spontaneous deliveries, N_2O-O_2 (6 and 3 litres respectively), with or without trichlorethylene (Trilene), using a non-rebreathing or semi-open system, is quite satisfactory. More recently methoxyflurane (Penthrane) with the same technique has been advocated. Both Trilene and Penthrane are excellent analgesics and can provide good anaesthesia for vaginal deliveries. Cyclopropane and oxygen in a closed system is still popular in many centres when deeper anaesthesia is required for difficult forceps deliveries. One must remember that cyclopropane and ether are flammable and explosive, and care must be taken to avoid sources of ignition including static electricity, which is a hazard with improper equipment and grounding procedures. Halothane (Fluothane), combined with N_2O-O_2, provides swift and smooth induction, and has replaced chloroform to produce uterine relaxation for version procedures. However, because halothane relaxes the uterus, prolonged or deep anaesthesia must be avoided.

Conduction anaesthesia The use of spinal anaesthesia is declining in Canada, and is being supplanted by the use of lumbar epidural (peridural, extradural) anaesthesia. Both of these methods of anaesthesia are excellent techniques for any type of delivery, but must be carried out with skill, full knowledge of their physiological effects on maternal circulation and respiration, and a co-operative patient. They should be undertaken only by trained physicians. The epidural route can provide prolonged analgesia and anaesthesia by the use of repeated injections through a sterile polyethylene catheter.

The earlier remarks on the foetal effects of anaesthetics must be remembered when choosing between general and conduction anaesthesia. There is some indication that the incidence of foetal depression is higher with general than with conduction anaesthesia. There is also a greater risk of maternal vomiting and aspiration under general anaesthesia. However, complications such as hypotension and the rare neurological complication can and do occur with conduction anaesthesia. Both forms of anaesthesia require much skill and patience. Conduction anaesthesia may increase the need for forceps during delivery, and requires time for its induction; hence it is more commonly used in the primigravida. General anaesthesia can be quickly applied, and is the more usual anaesthetic for spontaneous deliveries, particularly in the multigravida, and is the technique of choice for obstetrical emergencies.

Caesarean section Anaesthesia for Caesarean sections requires more inhalation anaesthetic, administered for a longer period, or a higher level of spinal or epidural anaesthesia with its attendant effects on circulation and respiration. The choice, as with vaginal deliveries, is a personal one depending on one's ability and experience. All things being equal, foetal distress and prematurity are better handled with conduction anaesthesia, whereas accidental haemorrhage and placenta praevia are better dealt with under general anaesthesia. Anaesthesia for elective caesarotomies may be general or conduction depending on the anaesthetist's preference. Generally speaking, preoperative sedation is omitted except for the use of belladonna drug (atropine or hyoscine) prior to general anaesthesia. Some anaesthetists induce anaesthesia with a small dose of thiopentone, not exceeding 150 mg in a 2.5 per cent solution. All inhalation agents have been used, but as some time may elapse between induction and delivery, light anaesthesia is to be preferred. Most anaesthetists prefer to intubate the patient after induction, and use moderate doses of relaxants (succinylcholine or d-tubocurare) to provide a balanced anaesthetic and muscle relaxation. Adequate manual ventilation must be carried out. Gallamine (Flaxedil), a popular muscle relaxant, is said to pass through the placenta and may cause foetal paralysis, and is consequently not recommended. During conduction anaesthesia, an anaesthetic machine must be at hand to provide oxygen or supplemental anaesthesia if necessary. Intravenous thiopentone or narcotic (meperidine) may be given after delivery.

COMPLICATIONS

The practice of anaesthesia for the pregnant patient is associated with a different set of hazards than those encountered in the elective prepared surgical patient and, therefore, must not be underestimated or undertaken without full appreciation of the potential complications and provision of the necessary equipment to deal with these complications when and if they occur. The flexibility and margin of safety are reduced in the administration of the depressant and potentially toxic drugs to pregnant women, particularly when they are in labour. These patients have a significantly increased blood volume, relative or actual anaemia, and a large abdominal mass which interferes with respiratory function, gastrointestinal motility, and cerebrospinal fluid dynamics. Finally, the infant's well-being both before and after delivery is largely dependent on the adequacy of maternal circulatory and respiratory functions.

MATERNAL COMPLICATIONS

Vomiting and aspiration Vomiting during labour is common, and aspiration of acid gastric contents, although uncommon, is hazardous and indeed may be fatal. Vomiting is more common in pregnant women who have eaten just prior to onset of labour, when gastric emptying has ceased, or in prolonged labour when gastric juices accumulate. The use of narcotics and general anaesthetics increases the incidence of vomiting, and with the suppression of the cough reflexes, aspiration may easily occur. Aspiration can only be prevented by the avoidance of general anaesthesia. The hazard may be reduced by the use of a gastric tube prior to anaesthesia or a cuffed endotracheal tube during anaesthesia. The increasing use of conduction anaesthesia attests to the anaesthetist's awareness of the hazards of general anaesthesia. A light general anaesthesia, skilfully applied, is still the choice of many anaesthetists, but it is carried out with the necessary equipment for suction and intubation immediately at hand.

The aspiration of acid gastric contents may lead to a condition known as Mendelson's syndrome, characterized by dyspnoea, cyanosis, bronchospasm, and hypotension. The clinical and X-ray findings are those of a widespread pneumonitis. Sudden death may occur because of acute cor pulmonale. Treatment consists of immediate intubation, suction, ventilation with 100 per cent oxygen, and the intravenous administration of hydrocortisone (100–500 mg), bronchodilating drugs (e.g. aminophylline), and an antihistamine. There is some evidence that this intense bronchiolar reaction is the result of histamine release. Treatment should be continued with antibiotics and further steroids for three to five days, and with oxygen inhalation if necessary.

Hypotension Sudden falls in maternal blood pressure are due to acute blood loss, sympathetic paralysis associated with conduction anaesthesia (spinal or epidural), or compression of the inferior vena cava from the pregnant uterus, particularly when the patient is lying supine on a hard delivery table. Hypotension from sympathetic blockade is due to the intradural (spinal) or extradural (epidural) block extending well up into the thoracic area. Treatment consists of the intravenous administration of a vasopressor agent.

The supine hypotensive syndrome can be easily determined and treated by placing the patient in the lateral position or manually displacing the uterus to the left.

Reaction to local anaesthetics Acute sensitivity to local anaesthetics is a rare occurrence. Most so-called reactions to local anaesthetics are due to the inadvertent intravascular injection of the agent during infiltration or attempted nerve block. The patient suddenly becomes pale, hypotensive, and may have a generalized convulsion. Treatment consists of stopping the injection and administering 100 per cent oxygen by mask, and the use of a vasopressor if necessary. The use of intravenous barbiturates is not recommended, unless the seizure does not cease after adequate ventilation and restoration of the blood pressure.

Neurological complications – nerve palsies and paraesthesiae – are uncommon following spinal or epidural anaesthesia, providing sterile equipment and aseptic techniques are used. Occasionally postpartum patients develop paraesthesia in the region of the lateral femoral cutaneous nerve, or obturator nerve paralysis, with no evidence of root involvement. These nerve involvements may well be due to pressure effects of the foetal head in the pelvis, or may follow a difficult forceps delivery in a small pelvis.

Foetal complications
Foetal complications of obstetrical anaesthesia reflect maternal changes in circulation and/or respiration from the effects of drugs administered for analgesia and anaesthesia. Respiratory depressants (analgesics) pass readily through the placenta, and if reinforced by general anaesthesia and a difficult labour, may result in respiratory depression of the newborn to the point of apnoea. Maternal hypotension from any cause may severely curtail placental circulation, or even cause complete cessation during uterine contraction, resulting in severe foetal hypoxia. If the foetus is premature or there are obstetrical reasons for foetal distress, the addition of depression, hypoxia, or hypotension may have catastrophic effects on the baby.

RESUSCITATION OF THE NEWBORN

The most reliable guide for the need of active resuscitation of the newborn is the Apgar score at one minute after the umbilical cord

Table I

Apgar ratings

	Rating at one minute		
	2	1	0
Respiration	vigorous	depressed	absent
Heart rate	over 100	under 100	absent
Reflex activity	withdraws legs, coughs	sluggish movements	no response
Muscle tone	vigorous movement		flaccid
Colour	pink	blue	pale

has been severed (Table I). A newborn baby who has an Apgar score of 6 or less requires some form of active resuscitation. The incidence of low scores in large series of cases is higher following general anaesthesia than with conduction or no anaesthesia (e.g. 14 per cent versus 8 per cent in live births). However, this is not necessarily an argument for conduction anaesthesia or against general anaesthesia, as there are many factors involved which are not related to the anaesthetic technique. It does indicate however, that physicians practising obstetrical anaesthesia must be prepared and able to apply immediate resuscitative measures to the newborn when indicated. These measures are listed in order, depending on the severity of the foetal condition and the lowness of the Apgar score.

1 Gentle naso-pharyngeal suction.
2 Oxygen by mask delivered from a suitable device with reducing valve and flowmeter. The oxygen tank pressure must be reduced to 50 lb/sq in., and a flow rate of 2–3 L/min is adequate.
3 Mouth-to-mouth breathing.
4 Careful intubation with a small rubber or metal endotracheal tube, without traumatizing the larynx. Mouth-to-tube breathing can be carried out.
5 Application of some form of intermittent positive pressure device, as long as the positive pressure is of short duration and does not exceed 15 mm Hg.

There is no place for the use of respiratory stimulants in depressed babies. If the respiratory depression is due to narcotics, a small dose (one-tenth adult dose) of a narcotic antagonist may be injected into the umbilical vein and continue with some form of respiratory assistance. A 'sleepy' baby from general anaesthesia will quickly wake up if some form of gentle assisted ventilation is carried out and hypoxia is not permitted to occur.

Cardiotonic drugs are not indicated except in desperate situations where there is no heart beat. In this situation, if it is thought that the heart has just recently stopped, closed chest cardiac massage using two fingers should be carried out, and 1 cc of 1/10,000 adrenaline may be given by intracardiac injection.

Following resuscitation, babies should be kept warm and if necessary in an oxygen enriched atmosphere. The temperature of a newborn quickly falls if he is allowed to lie on an uncovered table or crib, and hypothermia may account for continued depression. In the case of premature babies, because of the danger of the development of retrolental fibroplasia, oxygen should continue to be administered in the minimum concentration required to keep the baby pink.

SUMMARY

There is a place for all forms of obstetrical anaesthesia, and over-enthusiasm for one technique at the expense of another, as well as over-anaesthetization, is to be deplored. There is a place for an anaesthetist in the delivery room for two reasons; to administer anaesthesia if it is required, and, at least as important, to resuscitate the newborn and the mother if this should be required. These occasions cannot always be foretold, and hence there is all the more reason for anaesthetic coverage, even for normal, uncomplicated obstetrics.

T.J. McCAUGHEY

15
Special considerations in paediatric anaesthesia

Many anaesthetists are apprehensive about anaesthetizing small children. Indeed, the oxygen demands of the child are high, his reactions quick, and his airway precarious. Yet, though experience helps, there should be no mystique about paediatric anaesthesia. The principles of adult practice can be adapted to the child with good effect if due account is taken of the differences in physiology and psychology.

PHYSIOLOGY OF THE NEWBORN

The newborn infant has just gone through a period of rapid and enormous change. The changes in the circulation are brought on largely as the result of increased oxygenation with the first few breaths of life. It is significant for the anaesthetist that pulmonary distress and hypoxia can cause a reversion to a foetal type of circulation. It appears as if nature would make it difficult for the unfit infant to survive. The majority of infants do survive, and are healthy, though their physiological findings may not be normal by adult standards.

Respiration in the Newborn
At the moment of birth the arterial oxygen tension is about 50 mm Hg., which is low by adult standards. After the first few days it has

risen to 70 mm Hg. Arterial carbon dioxide tension is high at the moment of birth, usually around 50–55 mm Hg, but this falls after a day or two to a level which would be considered low by adult standards. It is interesting to note that this low arterial carbon dioxide tension is roughly the same as that of the pregnant woman at term, being about 30–35 mm Hg.

The respiratory rate is around 40/minute while tidal volume is 15–20 ml. Anatomical dead space is about 1 ml per pound body weight, as later in life, or about 6 ml in the usual newborn. Physiological dead space may be high. Venous admixture due to right-to-left shunting is marked. The source of this right-to-left shunting has not been clearly identified but it amounts to as much as 20 per cent of the cardiac output. For the adult, about 2 to 3 per cent of cardiac output would be considered normal.

Resistance to Hypoxia in the Newborn
The infant appears able to withstand hypoxia better than the adult. This resistance may be more apparent than real. Mental retardation as the result of birth anoxia does not appear for months or years, and a cause-and-effect relationship is impossible to establish. But if mere survival is taken as the point of comparison, then the newborn does appear to be hardier in the face of hypoxia than the adult. It has been shown that successive bouts of hypoxia in the newborn deplete the myocardium of glycogen, and that beyond a certain point the myocardium will then fail on the next onset of hypoxia.

There are two reasons why the newborn can be expected to withstand hypoxia. Coming from the 'Everest' of the womb, he has an oxygen dissociation curve suited to operating best at low oxygen tensions. He is also equipped with more than the usual amount of haemoglobin, about 18 gm per cent. At birth 80 per cent of the haemoglobin present is foetal in type. By two months about 50 per cent of the haemoglobin is adult, 50 per cent foetal in type. By four months only 10 per cent of the haemoglobin is foetal.

The anaesthetist must proceed as if the infant were no more resistant to anoxia than the adult. The same standards of oxygenation should be applied as in the adult. At the same time the premature infant is particularly prone to oxygen toxicity as shown most strikingly in retrolental fibroplasia. In any long procedure or when artificial ventilation has to be continued for a long time, as in the care of infants with the respiratory distress syndrome, careful monitoring of arterial oxygen tension is essential.

PRINCIPLES OF AIRWAY MAINTENANCE AND VENTILATION

The principles of airway maintenance and ventilation are basically the same as in adults. Certainly the airways are smaller and more precarious. In the newborn infant, for example, one frequently uses a tracheal tube with an internal diameter of 3.0 or 3.5 mm. This seems extremely narrow by adult standards, but controlled respiration can be maintained very well indeed through such tubes. One should remember that oxygenation and ventilation can be better maintained if the infant is quiet and not struggling. For this reason the paediatric anaesthetist tends to use muscle relaxants as freely as in adults to keep the infant quiescent, to reduce oxygen demands, and to facilitate ventilation. Great attention to detail and constant supervision are essential if one is to give a safe anaesthetic to a newborn infant.

BLOOD REPLACEMENT IN THE NEWBORN

The infant does not tolerate blood loss any better than the adult. The total blood volume of the healthy newborn is between 250 and 300 ml. The loss of 10 to 15 per cent of the blood volume is as serious for the infant as for the adult. In addition, the loss is more difficult to assess. Accurate measurement of blood loss is extremely difficult when volumes are small. The measurement of central venous pressure is quite impracticable. The margin for overtransfusion is narrow. Fortunately the myocardium of the newborn is quite strong, unlike the myocardium of the older adult which usually suffers from some acquired heart disease. In fact even in the presence of severe congenital heart disease the myocardium itself is frequently quite strong.

It is a good rule to give serious thought to replacing blood loss over 12 to 15 per cent of blood volume. Certainly if blood loss is continuing in an extensive and prolonged operation and is likely to exceed 20 per cent of total blood volume, then blood should usually be given. These principles can be translated into some simple guidelines. A blood loss of 5 ml per pound body weight is about 12 per cent of blood volume. Spread over an hour or so such a loss is tolerable in healthy patients. A greater loss over a shorter period of time more sharply indicates blood replacement, particularly if the loss is continuing.

Time is an important consideration and 30 ml can be lost rapidly in a small infant. In a few cases the author has allowed the infant with a preoperative haemoglobin of 20 gm per cent to lose more than he would allow in an adult. Fluid replacement must be as accurate as possible.

FLUID REPLACEMENT IN AN INFANT UNDERGOING SURGERY

The fashions of fluid replacement in surgery change. The current trend is towards generosity. There seems little doubt about the sequestration of some volume of fluid from the extracellular space. The amount of this sequestration depends on the site of surgery and its magnitude and duration. When a serous cavity like the peritoneum is entered and major abdominal surgery is performed on the bowel, for example, most anaesthetists probably believe some of the evidence that a considerable translocation of extracellular fluid occurs. A sizable part of the extracellular fluid is functionally lost by a shift into or around the site of surgery. There are arguments about the accuracy of measurements of these shifts. Enthusiasts replace projected losses vigorously with salt solutions, in addition to blood and maintenance fluid replacement. The more sceptical are more conservative with fluids. It does not seem to make much difference to most patients.

Some recent evidence suggests that the sequestration of extracellular fluid in surgery of the newborn is similar in proportion to the adult. Again there seems no need to take this as an absolute indication to give large volumes of fluid. However, the daily turnover of extracellular fluid is very high in the infant. If he comes to surgery fasted he is also frequently acidotic. For this reason some fluid should be given and, if necessary, buffers such as sodium bicarbonate to correct metabolic acidosis. The blood gases from a capillary sample of blood from a warmed extremity or ear will give a good idea of the respiratory and metabolic status. A simple regime for fluid replacement during and after surgery might be: 5 ml/kg/hr of a balanced salt solution (Ringer's) in addition to blood loss replacement. Maintenance for the first two postoperative days can be done with 40 ml/kg/24 hours. If a solution with the pH adjusted to 7.4 is used, some correction of metabolic acidosis will occur. If metabolic acidosis is thought to be marked it should be measured by blood gas estimations and corrected by sodium bicarbonate.

TECHNIQUES OF ANAESTHESIA IN INFANTS, ENDOTRACHEAL INTUBATION

This is easy to do in infant and child once one gets used to the sizes of things. To intubate, one must find the epiglottis. The epiglottis in the infant is small and rather easy to miss at first. With a little practice confidence is acquired. The larynx should be displaced posteriorly by an assistant's finger. This is the single most useful trick in intubation. The position of the head and neck are the same as in the adult. The infant has a large head in proportion to his trunk and a short, weak neck. When placed flat on his back there is some flexion of the neck on the trunk and the head can be tipped backward before insertion of the laryngoscope.

Awake intubation is taught by some paediatric anaesthetists. Some restraint by an experienced assistant is necessary. Bucking on the tube is minimal. Though the technique is useful it is unnecessarily traumatic. An easy intubation can be done after muscle relaxants, properly used. The most important thing to remember is to oxygenate the infant well for at least two minutes before injecting the relaxant. If this is carefully done then there is a comfortable period of at least one minute of apnoea permitted for intubation.

MUSCLE RELAXANTS IN INFANTS AND CHILDREN

Muscle relaxants are extremely useful drugs in infants and children. Those commonly used are succinylcholine, d-tubocurarine, and gallamine. A new muscle relaxant, pancuronium, is extremely promising, being apparently as effective as d-tubocurarine without its ganglionic-blocking side-effects.

Succinylcholine

Succinylcholine is a short-acting, depolarizing muscle relaxant very commonly used in adults but equally effective in infants and children. The intubating dose is 1 mg/3 lb body weight intravenously. This causes apnoea in 30 seconds and usually lasts three minutes or so. One can also intubate following intramuscular use of the drug, 1 mg/lb body weight, which may not have induced complete apnoea at the end of 60 seconds but still permits intubation at this time. Veins are sometimes hard to find in infants and this technique can be invaluable.

Prolonged apnoea with succinylcholine There are two causes of prolonged apnoea with succinylcholine. These are overdosage and genetic abnormalities of plasma cholinesterase. The depolarizing action of succinylcholine begins to change to a non-depolarizing, curare-like effect when one has given about three or four times the intubating dose. It is therefore not surprising that recovery from succinylcholine is slow when given by drip over some hours. It is therefore better to use curare for longer operations.

The other cause of prolonged apnoea from succinylcholine, genetic variation of plasma cholinesterase, is apparently never manifest in the newborn period. Nobody appears to know why. In fact the duration of action of succinylcholine in the newborn, on a body weight basis, is definitely shorter than in the older child. The probable reason for this is that the circulation to these areas is very active at this period of life, resulting in more rapid removal of the drug. When prolonged apnoea occurs in the child, his parents and relatives should be investigated for genetic variations of plasma cholinesterase. When an atypical plasma cholinesterase is discovered, the drug must be avoided on future occasions. The treatment of the prolonged apnoea is artificial ventilation until adequate spontaneous respiration returns.

Contraindications Succinylcholine ought not to be given to certain severely burned patients. These are patients with ungrafted third degree burns covering more than 20 per cent of the body surface area and of more than three weeks' duration. Cardiac irregularities and standstill follow the drug in these patients frequently enough to proscribe it. In these patients the drug causes a sharp rise in serum potassium. A similar rise occurs in patients with large areas of denervated muscle, as in paraplegics.

Since succinylcholine causes a rise in intraocular pressure it ought to be avoided in children with open penetrating eye injuries.

Malignant Hyperthermia
This is a serious complication of anaesthesia, particularly in children. In its fully blown form the syndrome is probably very rare indeed. Early recognition is the key to successful treatment. This complication is more fully discussed in chapter 12. Some paediatric anaesthetists monitor temperature in all children by a thermistor probe placed in the axilla.

d-Tubocurarine is a very useful drug in infants and children. In contradistinction to succinylcholine, the newborn shows an exaggerated response, rather like a mildly myasthenic patient. A dose of one milligram for each four pounds body weight will last for almost an hour. This dose will cause a drop in blood pressure in the adult, sometimes to an alarming extent. The cardiovascular system of the newborn does not seem so susceptible. In fact the drug is well tolerated and extremely useful, particularly in the very sick infant. In many of these sick infants very little anaesthesia indeed is given, perhaps 50 per cent nitrous oxide with 50 per cent oxygen. The infant is paralyzed instead with curare and artificial ventilation is maintained throughout. This can result in an immediate improvement in the patient's condition, allowing the anaesthetist to suck out the trachea if necessary and control ventilation and oxygenation.

INHALATION ANAESTHETICS IN INFANTS AND CHILDREN

The MAC in Infants and Children

MAC stands for minimal alveolar concentration. This is defined as the lowest alveolar concentration which will prevent movement on surgical stimulation in animals and man. The alveolar or end-tidal concentration relates closely to the anaesthetic concentration in the brain; but when there is poor ventilation-perfusion matching in the lung with an alveolar-arterial difference for the anaesthetic gas tensions, the alveolar concentration is no longer a faithful reflection of anaesthetic depth. Right-to-left shunting is the rule in the newborn infant, often to as much as 20 per cent of cardiac output at 24 hours of life, compared to about 3 per cent in the adult. Bearing these reservations in mind, researchers have measured MAC and found that it appears to decline steadily throughout life. In other words, it appears that the infant and child require a higher concentration of inhalation anaesthetic agents for a given depth of anaesthesia; and yet inhalation anaesthetics can be very dangerous, particularly in the infant. The reason for this is that the tidal volume in the infant is uneven and the uptake of the anaesthetic agent is accordingly somewhat unsatisfactory. The anaesthetist often resorts to artificial ventilation. The concentration of the anaesthetic agent can then be built up very rapidly to dangerous levels.

Halothane

Halothane is an extremely useful agent in children, but hazardous in infants. Cardiovascular depression rapidly follows artificial ventilation with halothane in infants. For this reason, particularly in the presence of congenital heart disease, halothane is not popular with neonatal anaesthetists.

In the older child halothane is very useful indeed. A total anaesthetic can be conducted without the need for intravenous agents. Induction can easily be done, provided one has the child's confidence, using nitrous oxide and halothane. Tracheal intubation can then be quickly performed and the child allowed to breathe spontaneously, or respiration can be artificially controlled if indicated. This technique is useful in practice and good for teaching residents simplicity and the principles of inhalation anaesthesia.

Hepatitis following halothane has caused much controversy. A cause and effect relationship has never been demonstrated, largely because the lesion in the liver is non-specific. The evidence against halothane has been entirely circumstantial. In any case hepatitis following halothane in children is rare indeed, the author not having seen a case in over 30,000 exposures, many of them repeated.

Other Inhalation Anaesthetics

Cyclopropane, a most useful induction agent, has fallen completely out of fashion because of its flammability. Other agents once popular and now completely ignored are ethyl chloride, divinyl ether, and diethyl ether. On occasion a despairing paediatrician will ask to have diethyl ether given for severe status asthmaticus. The theoretic indication here is nebulous, and in the hands of an anaesthetist most likely lacking experience and skill with this agent, the administration is certain to be difficult and dangerous.

As a maintenance agent methoxyflurane is useful when the surgeon wishes to inject epinephrine into tissues. Its slow uptake and excretion must be remembered.

THIOPENTONE

Some paediatric anaesthestists use thiopentone very frequently for the induction of anaesthesia even in small children or infants. The agent is given intravenously using a small needle. Momentary restraint by an experienced assistant is essential. The usual induction dose for adults, 3–4 mg/kg body weight, works well for children also. A simple rule is 1 ml of the usual 2½ per cent solution (25 mg) per year of life up to 10 years. Succinylcholine can then be given and the patient intubated. In skilled hands this technique is fast and impressive. If one misses or loses the vein it can be less elegant. Forcible restraint of a terrified child is tiring all around.

This technique causes apnoea at once and if the child has been breathing room air only and has been struggling, hypoxia can follow rapidly. I have never liked this technique personally except for larger children. Events follow each other rapidly after the use of two powerful drugs like thiopentone and succinylcholine. The sequence of physiological changes is impossible to demonstrate and to teach. This crash technique is nevertheless widely practised and taught in some excellent paediatric hospitals.

Thiopentone can be used with excellent effect in the older child. From about seven years of age onwards children will usually co-operate for an intravenous induction. It has to be done adroitly and a second try is not usually welcomed. From this age onwards anaesthesia can be conducted with the same techniques used for adults with only minor modifications.

MONITORING

The precordial stethoscope is the most important monitor in the child. An ordinary flat stethoscope ending is strapped over the precordium so that breath and heart sounds are audible. The diaphragm is not necessary and is best removed if frequent use is planned since it warps rather quickly. Paediatric anaesthetists have found ways of making the precordial stethoscope as servicable as possible, including monaural attachments and light, flexible tubing. Any stethoscope with a long extension will do.

The blood pressure should be recorded in every anaesthetic in a child or infant. There are small blood pressure cuffs which can be applied even to the arm of the newborn. If children are being treated in an adult hospital such special equipment may be lacking but a precordial stethoscope must never be omitted.

When major thoracic surgery is being done the circulation should be monitored by a central venous catheter and electrocardiography. On occasion electroencephalography gives a good idea of brain perfusion and oxygenation as when total heart bypass is in use. Some anaesthetists monitor body temperature continuously by a thermistor probe in the axilla. None of these devices should distract attention from the patient. The single most important one is the precordial stethoscope.

THE PSYCHOLOGY OF CHILDREN IN HOSPITAL

The newborn infant should, of course, be handled gently but there is no need for psychological expertise. The preschool child, the school-age child, and the adolescent are all somewhat different in their attitudes to their environment.

Separation from the mother at the age of two or three years, for example, is likely to be bothersome to both, in emergency circumstances. Happily, nurses in children's hospitals are particularly skilful at handling children kindly but firmly. The anaesthetist, or for that matter any other physician, can learn a great deal from these nurses. The nurse often gives the best clinical summary of the patient's condition and her evidence must always be treated with great respect. Indeed when looking over the patient's chart, it is not a bad idea to begin with the nurse's notes. Early and subtle changes are picked up and reported with remarkable precision by nurses.

The anaesthetist must be kind, good-humoured, patient but quite straightforward and firm. A certain amount of guile is useful. There is not much use in the man-to-man or let-us-keep-our-chins-up-and-be-brave approach. The preschool child may not be capable of understanding one's language. An atmosphere of unhurried kindness and understanding with a minimum of verbiage is essential. One should know the child's first name and use it naturally.

The school-age child is somewhat more likely to co-operate than his two-year-old brother. He is very sensitive to the atmosphere around him, and it should inspire confidence.

The adolescent is another story. Here the child is developing an awareness of his physical and mental self which he has not had till then. More detail may be needed in answering questions, but answers should still be simple.

The greatest satisfaction children afford their physician, of course, is their enormous power of recuperation. Their sickness passes away and is forgotten like a dream. The difference in atmosphere between children's and adult hospitals is striking. Children do not complain of their fate; adults consider sickness a personal affront and resent it.

EXAMPLES OF ANAESTHESIA FOR PAEDIATRIC SURGERY

Common Operations

Circumcision This is often done without anaesthesia a day or so after birth. If it has to be done some months later it is still usually considered a minor operation. The anaesthetic, though, is a major one. A tracheal tube should be inserted under succinylcholine given intravenously or intramuscularly. Respiration should be assisted and halothane is a useful agent here. A precordial stethoscope and blood pressure recording are minimum requirements for monitoring.

In all infants the recovery period is one requiring immediate supervision. At the moment when the tracheal tube is removed, to take the analogy of severing the umbilical cord after birth, the infant should have an Apgar score of 9 or 10, that is, he should be moving all four limbs, with a good tone, have a strong, rapid pulse of 120 to 140 per minute, be breathing adequately, and crying loudly. If the unconscious infant is left without a tracheal tube he quickly tends to develop obstructed breathing.

Hernia Repair A common operation performed with increasing frequency earlier in life. Tracheal intubation is much safer for the patient. Monitoring should include at least the use of a stethoscope on the precordium and blood pressure measurement. A scalp vein needle can be inserted in a small vein on the dorsum of the hand and a slow intravenous drip of 5 per cent dextrose in water run throughout the operation.

Tonsillectomy and adenoidectomy Probably one of the commonest and certainly one of the worst done operations. The anaesthetist is spared, luckily, the controversy over indications. A tracheal tube is essential. The surgeon and the anaesthetist jointly share the responsibility for the airway and complete understanding must prevail. This is a difficult anaesthetic requiring constant attention. If an inhalation technique is used for induction, for example with nitrous oxide, oxygen, and halothane, large adenoids and tonsils can obstruct the airway. The anaesthetic must be deep enough so that there is no swallowing or straining during the procedure. Halothane is quite satisfactory and respiration can be assisted with advantage. One should never underestimate the demands of this operation and anaesthetic. Again, the anaesthetist should constantly monitor blood pressure and heart and breath sounds. In the recovery room expert nursing care is needed.

Emergency surgery Aspiration of vomitus is still the greatest cause of preventable deaths under anaesthesia. It follows that one should be as sure as one can be that the stomach is empty before inducing anaesthesia. Six hours fasting from food and fluids is reasonable. On the other hand, if children are to be operated upon after midday one should expressly order fluids to be given six hours before surgery to prevent excessive dehydration and acidosis.

Fractures The commonest cause of dispute between surgeon and anaesthetist is over the optimal time to reduce fractures. Only children with those fractures where time is a critical consideration for recovery of function should be done as soon as possible, even if food has recently been taken. Open fractures and fractures involving loss of vascular supply to a limb or part of it, for example supra-condylar fractures with an absent radial pulse, must be treated as soon as possible. Regional analgesia, for example axillary block, should then be given first consideration. If general anaesthesia is unavoidable, and a meal has been taken within six hours, an attempt must be made to empty the stomach by using a wide-bore stomach tube. If this induces vomiting, so much the better. The anaesthetist will then proceed as if the stomach were still full.

Bleeding following adenotonsillectomy A very serious emergency, often underestimated. On occasion the child has been bleeding for hours before being returned to the operating room. One must take time, then, to assess the amount of fluid and blood loss. In many cases a litre of lactated Ringer's solution or 500 ml of blood will be needed before surgery.

In these cases there are always blood clots and fluid blood in the nose and oropharynx, and in the stomach. The stomach cannot be emptied adequately of particulate matter by suction tube. The anaesthetist must suck out the throat using a metal tonsil sucker, before induction. This may cause the patient to vomit and to empty his stomach. One may then proceed cautiously with the anaesthetic, inserting a tracheal tube under succinylcholine relaxation at the earliest moment.

Cuffed tracheal tubes are not commonly used in children and never in infants. If the child is over ten years of age a cuffed tube may be advantageous and may result in a much more airtight fit. Below this pre-adolescent stage, cuffs are seldom needed and are therefore needlessly traumatic. The larynx in the infant and child is narrow and deep compared with the adult larynx. Leaking is minimal even when tubes without cuffs are used. Cuffed tubes are ordinarily essential in adults.

Acute laryngotracheobronchitis and acute epiglottitis These two conditions are quite different in their clinical course and in the danger they pose to life. Acute epiglottitis is rapid in onset and rapidly obstructive. A tracheostomy should be done as soon as the diagnosis is made, that is, as soon as the swollen, red epiglottis is seen by cautious depression of the tongue.

Acute laryngotracheobronchitis comes on more slowly and is less rapidly asphyxiating. The vast majority of those with acute laryngotracheobronchitis can be managed in an atmosphere of maximum humidity with the use of intravenous steroids. Tracheal intubation has been used to tide patients over the period of a day or two while the airway is narrowed by swelling. The author has never been comfortable with this technique, preferring tracheostomy for those few patients who cannot be managed safely with humidity and steroids. In some centres patients with laryngotracheobronchitis have been successfully treated with racemic epinephrine given by an intermittent positive pressure inhaler. One centre claims to have virtually abolished the need for tracheostomy. This technique is useless for acute epiglottis which must always be regarded as a distinctly different condition.

In these cases the anaesthetist has the patient's life completely in his hands. Once the airway is secured by tracheal tube, an unhurried tracheostomy can be done. The best course here is to insert the tracheal tube while the child is awake. The swollen, inflamed epiglottis of acute epiglottitis can make this quite difficult.

The most important thing is to know when tracheostomy is indicated. In the case of acute epiglottitis this is as soon as the diagnosis is made. In the case of acute laryngotracheobronchitis the moment is more difficult to define. A rising pulse rate and signs of exhaustion are ominous. In any case the child must have continuous medical and nursing supervision as obstruction can occur very rapidly.

Pyloric stenosis This is the commonest operation, after circumcision, in the first two months of life. It should not be regarded as an emergency. Replacement of fluids and electrolytes must be done most assiduously. An isotonic saline drip is set up to replace sodium and chloride ions. The metabolic alkalosis, which may have existed for weeks, inevitably results in a loss of total body potassium which is much greater than that reflected by serum potassium. Potassium supplements must be given. A few days of intensive intravenous therapy may be needed to achieve reasonably normal serum electrolytes.

Congenital abnormalities Most surgery in the neonate is devoted to these problems. Some of these patients pose technical problems; for example, hare lips may occasionally be difficult to intubate, others require preoperative and postoperative intensive care. When the infant is very sick, as in the case of oesophageal atresia with tracheo-oesophageal fistula resulting in aspiration pneumonitis, surgery and anaesthesia are merely incidents in a prolonged period of special care. In all of these cases the anaesthetist relies heavily on the use of muscle relaxants (curare works well) and light anaesthesia.

In the case of congenital diaphragmatic hernia a special set of very difficult circumstances prevails, making intensive care absolutely essential. One leaf of the diaphragm is missing and some or all of the abdominal contents are in the thorax. The lung on that side is consequently much compressed or may be underdeveloped. The infant frequently needs intubation and resuscitation before coming to the operating room. Again only muscle relaxants and controlled respiration are needed. The anaesthetist and surgeon have a very difficult problem when abdominal closure is attempted. The abdomen has never held the usual contents and it may be impossible to close the peritoneum once the viscera are placed within it. A sheet of plastic material may need to be placed over the contents and stitched to the abdominal wall. The infant requires superb nursing and medical care postoperatively and certainly will need artificial ventilation for some days.

Congenital heart disease Infants and children usually withstand anaesthesia and surgery for congenital heart disease remarkably well. Open heart surgery is seldom performed under three or four years of life. Palliative surgery may be needed in the newborn to reduce pulmonary hypertension by partially occluding the pulmonary artery. This pulmonary band will have to be removed, and this is sometimes a little difficult, when total correction of the defect is done some years later by open heart surgery. Many operations, such as uncomplicated persistent ductus arteriosus, coarctation of the aorta, and closures of atrial and ventricular septal defects, carry very small mortality indeed, with modern hospital techniques.

Halothane is not favourably regarded as an agent for the small infant with congenital heart disease. In low concentrations it can be used with good effect to supplement anaesthesia in older children but most of the accent is on the use of muscle relaxants, particularly tubocurarine, and nitrous oxide and oxygen.

CONCLUSION

Paediatric anaesthesia demands a detailed knowledge of the physiological changes at birth and in the newborn, and of the pathophysiology of congenital abnormalities. The anaesthetist must understand the psychology of the child.

The principles applicable to adult anaesthesia hold good in children. These principles must be adapted from the point of view of technique and equipment. One must constantly pay attention to the airway. Monitoring must always include the precordial or oesophageal stethoscope.

The infant and child are excellent subjects for anaesthesia. Their naturally cheerful disposition and wonderful powers of recovery make them most rewarding patients.

Index